CRYSTALS FOR BEGINNERS

The Complete Crystal Reference Guide for Personal Healing

(The Unique Guide to Discover and Get Started With the Healing Power of Crystals)

Dennis Grajeda

Published by Harry Barnes

Dennis Grajeda

All Rights Reserved

Crystals for Beginners: The Complete Crystal Reference Guide for Personal Healing (The Unique Guide to Discover and Get Started With the Healing Power of Crystals)

ISBN 978-1-7751430-6-2

All rights reserved. No part of this guide may be reproduced in any form without permission in writing from the publisher except in the case of brief quotations embodied in critical articles or reviews.

Legal & Disclaimer

The information contained in this book is not designed to replace or take the place of any form of medicine or professional medical advice. The information in this book has been provided for educational and entertainment purposes only.

The information contained in this book has been compiled from sources deemed reliable, and it is accurate to the best of the Author's knowledge; however, the Author cannot guarantee its accuracy and validity and cannot be held liable for any errors or omissions. Changes are periodically made to this book. You must consult your doctor or get professional medical advice before using any of the suggested remedies, techniques, or information in this book.

Upon using the information contained in this book, you agree to hold harmless the Author from and against any damages, costs, and expenses, including any legal fees potentially resulting from the application of any of the information provided by this guide. This disclaimer applies to any damages or injury caused by the use and application, whether directly or indirectly, of any advice or information presented, whether for breach of contract, tort, negligence, personal injury, criminal intent, or under any other cause of action.

You agree to accept all risks of using the information presented inside this book. You need to consult a professional medical practitioner in order to ensure you are both able and healthy enough to participate in this program.

Table of Contents

INTRODUCTION 1

CHAPTER 1: ALL ABOUT CRYSTALS 4

CHAPTER 2: ANCIENT WISDOM & ESOTERIC KNOWLEDGE 16

CHAPTER 3: BENEFITS OF CRYSTALS AND STONES 32

CHAPTER 4: THE ORIGIN OF HEALING CRYSTAL 40

CHAPTER 5: MEANINGS OF HEALING GEMSTONES 57

CHAPTER 6: CLEAN AND CHARGE CRYSTALS WITH THE POWER OF EARTH, AIR, FIRE, AND WATER 75

CHAPTER 7: CRYSTSL SHAPES 102

CHAPTER 8: CRYSTALS FOR STRESS-RELIEF 112

CHAPTER 9: BLOODSTONE... 118

CHAPTER 10: MORE THAN 380 DIFFERENT CONDITIONS AND THEIR HEALING CRYSTALS 141

CHAPTER 11: HOW TO USE CRYSTALS FOR HEALING 162

CHAPTER 12: COMPLETE CRYSTAL FROM A TO Z 181

CONCLUSION... 203

Introduction

Are crystals magic? If not, then why are they popular? To all the students of the earth who want to connect to their crystals in a personal way, this book will guide you to your journey. Even Theophrastus—a meritorious Greek philosopher, and Pliny—a remarkable Roman geographer used crystals for their healing power. If you are fascinated about the colours of different types of crystals, or if your pupils dilate when you look at those colourful stones, or whether you just want to know about their mechanisms to heal your body, this book covers all. Unravel everything from coping up with anxiety to fighting the stress that is caused during your hard-working day. This book will take you to a journey where you will discover step-by-step ways to heal your body through crystals. You will get to know about every type of crystals and the detailed information on it ranging from unique, different properties. You will learn about how each crystal impacts an individual's mental health, spiritual health, physical health, emotional health, and psychological health. Crystals seem like a source of power. They are impressive in regards to any type of shape they carry. Mystery accompanies them.

If you want to cleanse your system and charge your system with positive energies, this book is for you. If you want to be more zen about your life via using crystals, this book is for you. If you want to know how to position your crystals in the right way, this book is for you. From creating harmony in your life to learning how to detox your body with the crystals, this book provides you everything. If you want to know about what type of crystals are right for you, this book is for you. If you want to know more about how crystals residing deep inside the earth carrying strong vibrations can tune your frequencies which are usually out of tune, then this book is for you. On the other hand, modern science is always for a lookout to find other ways for improvements whether to cure any diseases, or optimizing health, but there is nothing wrong with choosing another method to find out for yourself that if it works for you or if it doesn't work for you. So, if you are reading this book, take crystals as your guide and you will naturally discovery everything about crystals and their ways to improve your life efficiently and effectively. Some sources say that crystals hold within itself the power given to us by the Gods. So, read this book if you want to unravel the aura of their mystery.

Chapter 1: All About Crystals

What is Crystal Healing?

Have you stopped to imagine that crystals not only represent an element of nature? Through crystal healing, they have the power to transform health and generate benefits for all of us.

In the end, what is crystal healing? Learn the benefits of crystals for health in this exclusive book that I prepared for you. Are you one of those who likes to decorate the house with some crystals? It is natural that these beautiful colored stones are part of some corner of the shelf, making our home more harmonious.

However, crystals have a meaning and can be worth much more. Have you heard of crystal healing? It is a therapy where crystals are used as a main element to cure emotional and physical pain. The crystals act harmoniously, balancing our energy field due to their chemical and physical properties. They are so powerful that they charge an electromagnetic field with high vibrational power. The professional uses the crystals to perform an energy cleaning, providing the patient with improvements in health and well-being.

The use of crystals as an instrument of artistic vitality healing is called energy crystal healing. Here, healing is by the healing energy of the crystals focusing on the affected area of the body or the chakras in the human body.

Do Healing Crystals Actually Work?

If you enter the world of alternative medicine, you may have heard of crystal, some mineral names such as quartz and amber. People believe in their healthful properties. Holding crystals or placing them on the body is thought to promote physical, emotional and spiritual healing. It is said that the crystal does this by actively interacting with the energy field or chakras of your body. While some crystals should relieve stress, others are said to boost concentration or creativity.

Crystal Healing, an Ancient Therapy

Although it is still a novelty for many people, healing with crystals exists thousands of years ago when man began to observe and notice the power of crystals. They observed that the crystals could be used as a healing tool and since then, this therapy has become stronger and stronger.

Benefits of Crystals for Health

Well, before you know a little about the benefits of crystals in health, we need to talk about our body and its energies. Our body, in addition to the anatomical and physiological composition, has energies that directly influence our state. This energy system, when we are not feeling well, becomes weak and consequently an imbalance occurs.

Have you entered any environment and felt weird as if the energy of the place was heavy? So, it is common to have that feeling in some moments because we are suffering energy interference all the time. That is why a therapist who works with crystal healing needs to know very well the properties of the crystals and thus, use each stone according to the needs of the patient. Some, in addition to the use of

crystals, work with essences, florals, and other important elements that can balance the patient's energy:
Provides deep relaxation
Greater feeling of well-being
Help detoxify
Fight depression and stress
Help to fight the allergies
Relieves headaches and muscle aches
Help in vibrational elevation

Is Crystal Healing Linked to any Religion?

The answer is no. We know that many people prefer to seek alternative treatments and therapies and that they are not linked to any religious ideology. Crystal healing is not linked to any religion and its only mission is to work esoterically on healing and energy balance. The focus is only to work the energetic functions of the human body, which is formed by three main structures: energy fields, chakras and conductive energy channels.

Our aura is divided into seven energy levels; each of them has a type of frequency. In the case of the chakras, they act through our body tissues and it has the function of regulating our emotions. And in the third group, we have the energy channels, which have the mission of distributing the forces through our body. Perceive how everything is an energy system, being constantly influenced by our actions, thoughts, places we go through and diseases. Making positive and good energy is one of the functions of this crystal treatment!

How Do Crystals Work?

When a patient begins a treatment through crystal healing, the contact of the stone enters the energy system, thus resonating with the entire system. The result of this is the rebalancing of the energies and consequently of the emotions of that of well-being. Many patients report that after the end of the session, they feel lighter and more emotionally balanced.

Physical Illnesses

It is very important to emphasize that unfortunately, many times, our body gets sick. When it comes to a physical illness, it can be a spinal problem or even something more serious that needs a medical evaluation. In this case, the patient can continue with crystal healing. However, he must seek a specialist with the intention of receiving the necessary treatment for his case.

Crystal healing helps in recovery, with the main focus on restoring energy balance. This is, in fact, very beneficial when the patient is going through a more serious physical illness. But the patient should never refuse medical and professional help as well as deny the use of appropriate medications.

Basic Properties of Crystals

What is the most essential property of a crystal? Both crystals and chakra stones are known to have condensing energy on mass. Thus, a crystal can be used to absorb, store item and focus on the subtle energy. This can be better understood with the scenario below. Let us consider a possible rechargeable battery. It can be used to absorb, store and release electrical energy. The same crystal can absorb, store items and focus life energy.

Programmable

If we look at the perspective of natural crystals, we will see small sparks in light. These small sparks are the sparks of consciousness of light. This is a very basic form of consciousness. Natural crystals will have more sparks of consciousness and synthesis crystal. Therefore, natural crystals will be better than synthetic crystals and will be a better choice for crystal treatments.

Unlike humans, plants or animals, a crystal does not have any willpower because it does not have its own ideas. So it will follow any instructions without causing any resistance. If we say "absorb life energy", it absorbed life energy. If we say "project life energy", it will project life energy because people and animals have the ability to think. This gives them consciousness and willpower. That's why they may or may not follow every instruction. If we tell them what to do, they can resist. If we can control animals to do something, it may or may not obey us because it has willpower. Even plants are conscious. It has been discovered that when a person speaks to them, they tend to grow faster, bigger and healthier. Plants also have Willpower but to a lesser extent.

Chakra Activator

A crystal or chakra stone can also be used to activate the chakra. This means that the crystal can be used as a chakra activator. If we place it directly on the crystal chakra, the chakra gets activated. If the clairvoyant only needs to look at the chakra, it consists of after the crystal is activated, he will see that the chakras appear to be larger, rotate faster and have more energy. The crystal will not only be activated, but it will also activate the lower chakras.

Basic Techniques of Crystal Healing

There are four basic techniques of crystal healing for processing and utilizing crystals:

Cleaning is the process of removing dirty energy.

Charging is the process by which life energy is placed on the crystal.

Programming is the process of giving crystal instructions. This way, the absorbed energy will stay in the crystal.

The 10 Most Effective Healing Stones

1. Amethyst

Amethyst is a crystal that is known to be used to help cure hangovers and drunkenness. It is also said that this particular crystal is good to help people connect with their spirituality and also to improve their psychic ability. Amethyst Crystal can be especially good for people with the following signs of the zodiac: Pisces, Virgo, Aquarius and Capricorn.

2. Rose Quartz

This crystal is also known as the "crystal of love." This stone is commonly used to attract and maintain love, as well as to protect relationships. Rose quartz can likewise help heal your heart from disappointment and pain. Rose quartz crystal can be particularly good for people with the following signs of the zodiac: Libra and Taurus.

3. Iron Pyrite

Iron pyrite can be used to prevent any negative energy or any physical danger you may face. This can likewise help activate your intellect and your memory even more. Iron pyrite crystal can be particularly good for people with the following signs of the zodiac: Leo.

4. Eye of Tiger

This crystal can be used to maintain and increase wealth. The Tiger Eye is also known for helping to create understanding and awareness; it can likewise be an excellent stone to use when you feel stressed, to keep calm. The tiger eye crystal can be particularly good for people with the following signs of the zodiac: Capricorn.

5. Hematite

This particular crystal is often used to land and balance in your life. It can be an amazing stone to have if you are under stress and need to feel calm and focused. This crystal can also help clear any negative feelings that arise from stress or anxiety. Hematite crystal can be especially good for people with the following signs of the zodiac: Aries and Aquarius.

6. Raw Emerald

This is another crystal that can help with love. This crystal is often referred to as the stone for "successful love." This crystal can promote focus, eliminate negativity and foster loyalty and sensitivity. Raw Emerald Crystal can be especially good for people with the following signs of the zodiac: Taurus, Gemini and Aries.

7. Citrine

Citrine crystal is often used due to its warm and optimistic energy that it can emit and also has the additional advantage of not having to be cleaned or recharged. This crystal also helps repel any negative energy that crosses your path. Citrine Crystal can be particularly good for people with the following signs of the zodiac: Gemini, Aries, Libra and Leo.

8. Celestina

Celestine crystal can be ideal for calming and balancing. Some persons who have used this crystal have said it helps them remember their dreams. Celestina can also help provide clarity and peace to your body. Celestine Crystal can be especially good for people with the following signs of the zodiac: Gemini.

9. Quartz Crystal

Quartz stone is a crystal that has a source of pure and powerful energy. This Crystal can help you feel more conscious, as well as stimulate your brain and make you feel more active and at alert. This crystal could be an excellent stone to use if you feel tired mentally and physically. Quartz crystal can be particularly good for all signs of the zodiac.

10. Desert Rose

This crystal is sometimes used during meditation, as it has been said to be used as access to past and future lives. It can bring about mental clarity, as well as perception and knowledge to the owner of the crystal. The Desert Rose crystal can be especially good for people with the following signs of the zodiac: Taurus.

Chapter 2: Ancient Wisdom & Esoteric Knowledge

Subtle Energy, Vibration, and Frequency
As mentioned at the end of Chapter 1, all life on earth has a spiritual-energetic element. You are already aware that crystals are influenced by astrological activity and the planets and that they too have a spiritual-energetic energy to them. Everything in the universe can be said to work on a law of vibration and frequency. In other words, everything is interconnected, intrinsically connected through time and space. There are so many factors which can influence this time and space. The mind for one is a powerful tool. It can create, destroy, affect and influence. The mind can re-shape, re-structure and, on some level, alter subatomic particles through the thoughts and intentions emitted alone. Now, this has some fascinating implications, especially when wishing to start harnessing the healing benefits of crystals.

If the mind has such a powerful effect to influence physical reality, then imagine what we can do with a crystal already pre-programmed and metaphysically charged! As we will explore in more detail later, we can harness the power of our minds through the natural law of vibration and frequency to enhance the qualities of the crystal, which then further amplifies its healing effect on us. Essentially, we can charge crystals with the power of our thoughts and intentions.

Scientists and quantum physicists have discovered some amazing things regarding the law of frequency and vibration and the power of our minds. Not only are our thoughts powerful influencers and shapers and creators of reality, but they also can be used to change the course of an action and future goals and create parallel universes. That is correct; our minds can create alternate realities! There was an experiment conducted called 'the double slit experiment.' Scientists recorded the effect of an observer on subatomic particles traveling towards a screen.

Without going into too much detail, they found that the presence of an observer, i.e. the human eye (observation), actively changed the course and direction of the subatomic particles. Furthermore, there has been much research discovering that we can change the molecular structures of plants, water, and our own cells from the thoughts we project.

In this sense, our thoughts are literally projectors of the world around and within, shaping and creating as we perceive. So, when it comes to crystals which have been formed through vast amounts of energetic pressure and astrological influence from the elements and planets, we ourselves are the deciders of whether we wish to be open to the magical benefits of the crystal queen and kingdom. Just like a current which requires a full circuit to work, the mind holds great power to open and receive all the various wonders of crystals, or to close oneself off either through, fear, disbelief, or unwillingness to evolve.

Our Subtle Bodies

This brings us onto the subtle bodies of man. The subtle bodies of man- or woman- are energetic layers constructing the whole self. Just as the earth is a living conscious entity designed to achieve wholeness, balance, and equilibrium, we humans are complex. Our bodies are designed to achieve homeostasis, yet we are not just the physical body. Our self- the whole, balanced and integrated self- consists of many bodies. These bodies are all equally significant, merging together to create the whole. Subtle energy is in everything, from the food we eat to the air we breathe. Subtle energy essentially flows through every living thing and it is subtle energy which allows crystals to heal us and raise our vibration.

So, before we proceed onto how they do this; what are the subtle bodies of man? The key is to be mindful of why we are exploring the layers of ourselves and how they can relate to our journey of healing and wholeness. Being aware of the interacting parts that make up our whole being can help us understand the nature of crystals better and we can further tune in and connect to their energy for our benefit. So, let's explore the subtle bodies of man and woman whilst keeping in mind the benefits, exercises, and techniques of connecting to them, which we will be exploring later.

The Aura

The aura is our protection. In Greek, aura is derived from the word meaning 'breeze,' and it is significant to keep this in mind when learning about your own aura. Just as every living thing has its own electromagnetic force or energy field, so do we. The aura is essentially this, an electromagnetic field of energy which surrounds our physical body, transmitting and receiving with interacting vibrations. Everything is vibration as you are aware as everything consists of a frequency. It is through the aura where we can pick up, be open to, and receive the positive energy of others and the natural world such as crystals, plants, and herbs, and it is also where we can protect ourselves from those energies, thoughts, and intentions which may wish to harm. This is one of the main intentions of the aura; it protects you from harmful energy.

As everything works on a law of vibration and frequency, if we have a weak aura and allow destructive energy in, this, in turn, affects all our other bodies. This is because the mind, body, and spirit are designed to work in harmony. Ultimately, the aura is the link to all the other subtle bodies of man. Any message or signal transmitted therefore has a profound effect on all aspects of being such as the astral, etheric, physical, mental, emotional, and spiritual bodies (we explore these next). This is why it is so important especially when opening yourself up to the powers of crystals and subtle energy, to protect yourself and engage in aura strengthening and protection exercises. We go through these in detail in the final chapter.

The Etheric Body

The etheric body is the energetic replica of the physical body. Any physical ailment, disease or distortion of the mind that arises occurs on the ether (in the etheric body). It is also through the etheric body where crystal healing occurs. Fundamentally, as all the bodies are connected and subtle energy is a forever flowing mix of subatomic particles, impressions, intentions, and vibrations, crystal healing is not exclusively equated with the ether. It is, however, important to remember it as a primary connection and link, mainly due to the connection between the physical body and the etheric body. Crystal healers, and yourself once you have learned and mastered the art of healing with crystals, can use crystals to disperse blocked energy on the ether, having a restorative effect and bringing harmony and balance back to your life force energy (chi, the universal life force). Thus, any ailment or illness is treated at the root cause, having a profound effect on all the other levels of being.

The Astral and Emotional Body

The astral and the emotional body are closely linked and some even suggest they are the same. This is because emotion comes from the word emote, which means to 'move out.' The astral body extends just beyond the etheric body and this is where emotions are usually felt and projected. Crystals, as we will explore later, can be used to heal and release emotional blockages on the astral layer, thus clearing energy pathways for improvement in all other areas of life. The astral and emotional bodies are particularly effective for healing repressed emotions or feelings and can also remove any distortions on the mental plane.

The Mental Body

The mental body essentially consists of the lower mind and the higher mind. It is also referred to as the lower self and higher self. This is because the self is essentially the mind. The mind is everything; it is consciousness. Using crystals to remove blockages, release repressions, and cultivate energy, therefore, activates consciousness in a way unique and synergistic to vibrational qualities of the individual crystal. Crystals have an electromagnetic energy field just as we do. Through consciously opening oneself up to harness their healing energy, through setting strong intentions and engaging in physical exercises to create a connection, one can receive and tune into the vibrational frequencies through the mental plane. As the mind is closely linked to all the other bodies such as emotions, this can, of course, be used to incredible advantage.

The Spiritual Body

The spiritual body is connected to the third eye; the seat of knowledge, wisdom, and intuition. This is where we perceive subtle energy. High idealism, morality, universal values like compassion and unconditional love, creative inspiration and advanced artistic and imaginative expression all come under the spiritual body's realm. The spiritual body essentially enables us to see, view and perceive the world in an interconnected way. It has strong links to the divine and higher aspects of consciousness. Knowledge and illumination of who we are on a deeper and soul level can be discovered through the spiritual body, and it is often where those who achieve enlightenment or self-mastery discover themselves. Fortunately for us, there are many crystals which work directly on the spiritual level that can help us access the divine and higher consciousness. They simultaneously alleviate blockages and release distortional frequencies along the way.

Elemental Energy

Just like astrological influences, the elements of nature have intrinsic and integral effects on the formation and healing qualities of crystals. It is important when exploring the influence of the elements that you take into account its effect on crystals. Crystals usually embody the qualities of an element, either earth, air, fire, water, or ether. In Chapters 4 and 5 we go through the individual crystals in detail, however, for now, let's explore the metaphysical and energetic properties associated with the elements.

Earth Energy

Earth is grounding. Crystals which embody a strong earth energy usually bring stability, grounding, organization, structure, and a sense of protection. They can aid in increasing feelings of duty, responsibility, practicality, and often enhance physical strength. This subsequently links to the mind and emotions. Crystals strong in earth energy can be connected to and harnessed to balance out any of the other elements. For example, say you are strong in water and a bit too sensitive, overly-emotional, or dreamy. Connecting to an earth stone can really help ground you and bring some needed structure back into your life. The same is true for if you are particularly fiery. Fire is great - it is passionate, expressive and can bring great joy, excitement, and creative passion and ambition for life. Yet too much of this may paradoxically prevent you from living your dreams and achieving success. An earth gemstone, therefore, would bring the practicality, grounding, and organization you require.

This energy helps you on a physical level, as you receive earth energy from the food you eat which contains minerals, vitamins and trace elements that are essential to the body. You need to align one's energies with the earth in order to maintain centered and motivated to help you follow your path in this life. Earth qualities are deepening, focusing, stabilizing and keep you centered. Earth stones help you keep your feet on the ground, and practically minded. Cornelian, chrysoprase, lapis lazuli (earth/fire), jade (earth/air), smoky quartz, bloodstone (earth/fire), garnet and all red stones all have earth energy.

Air Energy

Air energy is purifying and uplifting. It can bring feelings of lightness and being connected to spirit and subtle perception. Crystals strong in air energy often relate to communication, expression, and speech. For anyone struggling with writing and communication, or for someone who wishes to enhance their voice in any way, using air strong gemstones would aid greatly. In addition to its link to communication, air energy is also closely linked to intuition and connecting to the higher self (the higher mind). All forms of intellect, cognitive thinking and processes, and mental stimulation is associated with air, therefore air elemental crystals are often popular with deep thinkers, writers, those engaged in study and learning, scholars, poets, and philosophers. Some air strong crystals can also bring great creative expression, imaginative enhancements, and inspiration.

Air energy raises one's vibrations to the spirit. Air uplifts and purifies. We all know how we take in prana or life-force energy through our breath, we can breathe in these cosmic forces. Air energy assists in spiritual growth when an individual feels out of touch with their intuition or higher self. Amber, amazonite, amethyst, citrine, topaz, turquoise (earth/air), moss agate, moldavite, purple fluorite, emerald, diamond (air/fire) are all examples.

Fire Energy

Fire is passion, excitement, and inspiration. Crystals with fire energy are uplifting, purifying, expansive, stimulating, and can often bring creative expression and inspiration. Fire is essentially your life force, the universal energy responsible for vitality, energy, and will (action). Fire can be used to balance the sensitive and emotional nature of water, bring inspiration and optimism to the intellect and intuition of air, and add an extra oomph to the detailed and structured plans of earth. People strong in fire energy often have great passion and zest for life, however, may not be so in tune with the emotional, intuitive, and spiritual realms; such as those strong in water. Being knowledgeable of the healing powers of crystals, therefore, can greatly help with this.

By merging with the fire energy of a stone, one learns to focus on the life-force energy. This gives one power that we need to learn to use with wisdom. Fire qualities are purifying, stimulating, expansive and action-oriented. Crystals include ruby, obsidian, opal, peridot, rutilated quartz, sapphire, tiger's eye, pyrite, fire agate.

Water Energy

Water energy is intuitive, emotional, and yin in nature. Yin essentially represents flow, adaptability, emotional connection and wisdom, and the ability to navigate life with ease, calm, and grace. Crystals strong in water energy can aid intuition, develop heightened sensitivity, and bring emotional calm, balance, and serenity. Due to its strong link to intuition, water stones can be used for any activity related to creative, artistic, or imaginative expression and can also be connected to enhance spiritual and psychic qualities. This is due to water's association with the subconscious. Water as an element connects us to the subconscious, further allowing us to explore the shadow aspects of life, hidden emotions, feelings, impressions, and energy currents. This is essentially where it gets its intuition from. People strong in water are often emotional, sensitive, adaptable, and artistically or imaginatively gifted, and they usually have a direct connection to intuitive, psychic, and spiritual levels of subtle perception. Water gemstones can fine tune these sensitivities.

Our body is made up of over 70% water, so water energy has a strong effect on our energy fields. Herbal baths and swimming strengthen these fields, while water also cleanses and purges our emotions. Water qualities are flowing, surrendering, harmonizing, and accepting. Water governs the emotions and stones relating to the water element and help us integrate with one's higher self through the emotional body. Aventurine, aquamarine, calcite, moonstones, pearl, opals, coral, tourmaline, sugilite, rhodochrosite, rose quartz (water/earth).

Chapter 3: Benefits Of Crystals And Stones

Agate-This crystals will activate your faith, stimulate your internal talents, unleash your imagination and encourage you to think and evaluate more effectively. In addition to alleviating stresses and worries, Agate will allow you to succeed in all respects.

Amber-This mighty crystal takes up all negativity around you and replaces it with positivity-these forces allow the body to heal itself. Amber is also a very strong Feng Shui treatment for your anxiety for those who have suicidal feelings.

Amethyst — This stone will make your mind clearer and your attitude calmer, so your imagination and your information will run. It is an ideal Feng Shui therapy for those suffering from insomnia and frequent hallucinations because it will promote peace and peace of mind.

Aquamarine — The benefits of this crystal will benefit those who have difficulty expressing their feelings and speaking loudly. You will develop self-confidence and perseverance by repressing their anxieties and calming them. Aquamarine is a good time to use during experiments and meditation.

Aventurine — This crystal is very useful for focus and concentration, enabling quick decision-making and increased creativity flow. Therefore, your ability to lead others will be strengthened, and you will be able to overcome obstacles.

Bloodstone — In addition to being an excellent blood cleanser, this magic stone has the power to protect you from evil spirits and to suppress malicious thoughts.

Carnelian — This stone can promote perseverance, confidence, imagination, and leadership for those searching for the resources for advancing life so that you can better evaluate and appreciate the circumstances in your world.

Charoite — This rock is an effective Feng Shui cure for those who experience obsessive acts and compulsions. It also represses pressure by increasing any negative energy in your life and revitalizing your chi. Used Charoite leaves you happy and restless.

Clear Quartz — This lovely crystal has a strong force that can in many ways transform heat. It will also shield you from those who want to hurt you and cause you sorrow.

Garnet — This stone is a symbol of love, passion, and well-being. This removes any depression and stress in your life and increases your feelings of desire, attraction, and intimacy, helping you to feel closer and happier.

Hematite — This crystal, owing to its capacity to rejuvenate body oxygen and improve circulation, is highly regarded as a physical healer, by stimulating the absorption of iron by red blood cells.

Jade — This stone has been long wanted in ancient China for its ability to heal and protect. This pillar, a symbol of the beautiful and pure soul, will also provide mental clarity and a stronger flow of intelligence and creativity.

Jasper — This stone is a good cure for those suffering from headaches, migraines, and anxiety, it will relax their minds and promote relaxation, helping them to release their anxieties and feel more at peace with their souls.

Lapis Lazuli — This crystal symbolizes a strong spirit, as it strengthens your sense of adventure and helps you to feel more relaxed about your own life. Therefore, your fears will be diminished and you will see the world more clearly.

Moonstone — This branch, most often used as a Feng Shui treatment for women, addresses many of the issues they face: time cramps, menopause tension, and fertility barriers. Therefore, females who are using the Moonstone enhance their feminine qualities, activate internal instinct and become more physically attractive.

Obsidian — This stone is the perfect Feng Shui therapy for those who have low self-esteem and need improved confidence. Therefore, it's the perfect protection against negative chi in your life and defends you from people with evil intentions.

Onyx — The Onyx stone is a great Feng Shui cure for those who have recently got out of difficult relationships and are trying to move on. It will also maintain negative energy and keep the outlook optimistic and happy.

Peridot — This stone is commonly used by those who want to transcend the past, to let go of revolts and ancient feelings. Your heart will be free, clean, and no anger, envy, or wrath will be new.

Prehnite — This stone will ensure you are prepared for any scenario. It is also called the "unconditional love" rock and can heal any injuries and emotional problems. Therefore, Prehnite will increase your intuition.

Rhodochrosite — This stone, in Feng Shui, is a symbol of love and romanticism and continuous intercourse. It is also used to boost self-esteem and psychological needs for people who suffer from depression or denial following tragic events.

Rose Quartz — Known as the 'Love Stone,' this lovely product helps people with all kinds of romanticism, helps people pursue their partner in life, increases their long-term relationship value and fixes broken hearts.

Ruby — A crystal that revitalizes life, this brand brings joy to those who are searching for a greater purpose and fulfillment in their undertakings. It will help you to achieve your goals and ambitions and protect your assets against robbery or loss.

Rutilated Quartz — This stone has properties that substitute optimistic and romantic feelings with sadness, insomnia, remorse, and sad feelings. As a result, Quartz Rutilated has the potential to rekindle friendships and create a new sense of hope and imagination.

Saphire — This crystal, which is known as the "rock of wisdom," induces just that; a sense of mental clarity that removes all negatives and gives you a new mentality. Although Sapphire usually reduces mental stress, Sapphire blue is known to intensify the love emotions.

Smoky Quartz — This crystal is a good remedy for those who are lazily and lethargically impaired. By removing electromagnetic smog, an electromagnetic field that has dangerous effects on some, it creates a more focused and common-sense environment.

Sodalite — This stone helps people to discover and communicate their inner truths and stand by them regardless of circumstance. It is also a useful pillar for removing all electromagnetic fields, especially those generated by technology.

Tiger's Eye — Those who use the Tiger's Eye experience a new life drive and seek success. Through strengthening your faith, commitment, determination, and positivity, you will take your passion and make it happen.

Turkish — Many uses this lovely crystal to revitalize their chi and to create a sense of harmony. Turkey is also a cure for broken ties, building trust and hope. Use this stone to better communicate with your people.

Watermelon Tourmaline — Using this stone will help you to cope with compassion and flexibility for those who want to find new loves and embrace a relationship. You will also love yourself more and feel more joy and peace.

Zoisite — This crystal is an effective remedy for those with lethargy and depression; it reduces anxiety and encourages constructive energy. Therefore, you can achieve greater focus and imagination by using Zoisite.

Chapter 4: The Origin Of Healing Crystal

The History of Healing with Stones and Crystals

9,000 years ago, people were using crystals and gemstones to prevent illnesses and build jewelry and amulets to honor and worship their Gods. 5,000 years ago, Egyptians were crushing gemstones into powder and wearing it as makeup and to open up the intuition and the third eye, as well as to adorn the body in to help balance health and well-being. Today, people are studying crystals for their healing properties and utilizing them for a variety of healing purposes.

Considered a pseudoscience by modern medicine, the history of healing with crystals dates' way back to a time when modern medicine was unheard of and the local witch doctor was more likely to give you an herbal concoction and a crushed turquoise to eat with your daily bread. Toda, prescription medication tends to be the ruling classification of what works to aid the body without regard for the heart, soul, and spirit.

Together with a wide variety of other resources, the crystal or gemstone has been welcomed into more 'New Age' circles as being of great healing benefit to all levels of the self. Little research has actually been done by scientists to study the healing powers of the 'rocks' and it is unfortunate considering how well they work in collaboration with other healing methods and modalities

Right now, in our culture, people are looking for new ways to support their wholeness, not just their physical health. Many different tools are used in these 'alternative medicines' and can offer a higher vibrational frequency to any person who spends any length of time with a crystal or stone.

During the Roman Empire, the use of crystals and gems was widely known, possibly carrying over from the Egyptian Dynasties and had used in health, but were also considered for spiritual uses.

Roman soldiers were said to have rubbed crushed hematite on their bodies to make them 'invincible' on the battlefield. Other aspects of the same gemstone were used for drawing wealth and abundance to the wearer.

As early as 30,000 years ago, people were adorning their bodies with pieces of amber and lapis lazuli, buried with them in gravesites to indicate the importance of such sacred Earth gems. Even evidence dating BAC 60,000 years shows that we have held these articles and carried them with us throughout the ages.

Until the appearance of writing and cuneiform, there was hardly a way to understand exactly what these early humans were using their gemstones for, but since the time of the Ancient Sumerians and Egyptians, we have been better able to ask the questions about what each type of crystal meant to the health of the people using them.

It was noted in some ancient texts and discovered by archaeologists, that some Egyptians were buried with a Quartz

Crystal on their forehead to help them see better in the afterlife. Practices of mummification were not written about until sometime around 3500-3000 BCE. At this time, gemstones and their uses were also being written about, the same way that 'healers' were writing about the healing properties and uses of certain plants, flowers, and herbs.

Throughout history, there has been some kind of connection to how these crystals and stones were utilized, not just for adornment and the display of wealth and power, but to also align the wearer with specific healing energy or to repel or draw energies. All of the crystals and gemstones that we can account for today are also known to have some kind of healing property. These properties are not limited to the health of the physical body and are also connected to the wellness of the ethereal body, or spiritual essence, mind, and heart.

Descriptions of these types of properties began to arise at the time of the Ancient Sumerians and Egyptians and were possessed by those who were able to assess their qualities and offer them as aid and assistance to those in need of healing, almost like a herbalist would offer a bag of dried seeds or plant materials to someone looking for a remedy.

It is said that the ancient Grecian tale of Dionysius connects strongly to the properties of the amethyst stone and that its Greek name means "not drunken." This purplish crystal has been named this from an ancient time and in today's world has continued use as a stone to help with breaking addictions and remaining sober.

Many other stones were named for Greek words, including the word 'crystal', from the Greek 'krystallo', which meant ice, or glass. The clear quartz crystal appears as a shard of ice that never melts and so it was named by the Greeks.

The properties of the Quartz are numerous and it has been used as a general healing stone, as well as a tool of connection to the divine. There are several different varieties of Quartz that each have different properties and qualities and are called by different names.

The history of healing with crystals and stones is vast and long and the ways that these magical, earth energies were used are lost to time, but today we have continued to circulate the ancient knowledge of how to use these gifts and tools so that others can keep working with them for a healthier life and higher vibrational frequency.

It was sometime in the 1980s when a New Age of medicine and beliefs were being talked about and published more frequently. Books about crystals and alternative healing methods were seeing new light and there was a new dawn of crystal healing information that has continued to spread and become popularized by the internet and several different kinds of forums.

Even if you take a college course in geology you will be learning important data about the healing energy of these stones. They are made through pressure and time in the Earth's surface and are 'grown' all over the world. They have geometric formations that cause them to look and behave a certain way and all of these characteristics directly relate to the way they are used in healing practices. The more you know about them, the better.

The Energy and Vibrational Frequency of Crystals

Everything in our world is made of energy. All of us have a variety of energetic frequencies that we resonate with throughout the course of a day and a lifetime. Because we are all energy and have a system of energy centers within that resonate a vibrational frequency, we are able to connect to other energies of the same frequency easily. What's more, our energy can shift frequencies when we encounter things outside of ourselves that are either negative, positive, or neutral.

What do I even mean when I say frequency? A frequency is an imprint of energy, like a wave of a vibrational feeling. Here's a good example of what I mean: you set your hand on top of a computer monitor, it hums and you can feel its vibration. You are feeling the energy of electrical current speeding through all of the components inside to make that computer run.

Here's another example: when you hear a baby crying you feel the energy of that cry deeply, even if it isn't your child. It could be incredibly loud and obnoxious to you or it could inspire an urge to help the baby feel better, but either way, those reactions are both responding to the energy frequency of the crying emoted by the baby.

We all have the capacity to 'switch gears' in the moment and energy is the main ingredient in how we change course. Like a crystal, our natural resting state is a specific frequency or vibration of energy. When our energy is disturbed by an influence, like a cold or sickness, or perhaps the negative attitude of a customer at work, our entire energy system shifts and incorporates the energy of the illness or the bad attitude and we adjust to 'feel' that frequency instead of our original vibration.

Get the picture yet? To explain the vibrational frequency of crystals, it helps to know and understand that everything has a vibration and energy that it emits. What we do with that energy is up to us. Consider then the history of healing with crystals. It was obvious to ancient tribes and civilizations that there was more to a crystal or gemstone than just being pretty to look at. There were noticeable energies at work and they could be felt almost instantly.

Have you ever gone to a gem shop in your town? There are usually a couple that specializes in crystals, rocks, gemstones, and fossils and you should be able to find an eccentric and wide variety of each to look at and enjoy. When you walked inside did you notice the energy? If you picked up any of the crystals, could you feel it's frequency in the palm of your hand?

If not, that's okay. Sometimes, people are already just naturally more open to receiving or feeling the energy of objects. If you did, then you noticed that there is a clear difference between you and the crystal and that it is emitting some kind of energy. The reality is that the crystal you hold in your hand is being felt by your energy as you hold it.

How much have you already learned about chakras?

The seven chakras are a pillar of energies that reside within the matrix of your body and are connected to your physical organs and vital systems, your mental state, your emotions, and your spiritual well-being. All of these systems are energy. With the chakras connected to everything in your being, you will feel it on all levels when they become blocked and unbalanced.

The chakras go from the base of your spine (root chakra) to the top of your head (crown chakra). Each chakra has a different placement, qualities, properties, color, and vibrational frequency. Each one resonates at a different level and will be easily affected by the energies of each other as they work as a system, and by outside influences like environment, people, situations, life events and dramas, daily routines, the onset of illness, and more.

People are often using yoga practices, acupuncture, massage, and Reiki to heal their chakra imbalances, as all of these healing methods are known to heal and transform frequency and vibration. Crystals are also a popular tool because of how they radiate certain vibrations of energy to help your chakras find a better balance and healthier alignment.

Crystals and gemstones are created over time through the presence of certain elements, mixed with water and other minerals to form a solid structure. Some crystals and gems are found buried deep in the mountains and caves and must be mined for, while others naturally occur in visible places in the rocks on the surface. The elements themselves are naturally either crystalline or amorphous and will have either smooth edges because of repeating molecular patterns, or as with the amorphous stone, they will have more irregular patterns that cause the more rounded surfaces.

Many gemstones are cut and polished before they are sold so that they have a more rounded, shiny finish, but in general they tend to have a rougher exterior. Crystals often come in shards and are more frequently found 'as is' when you buy them or stumble upon them in their natural habitats.

Among the many crystals and gemstones that we have found and decided to make a part of our system of healing, there is none as powerful as the Quartz crystal. Quartz has, in fact, continued to be used in a variety of electrical engineering practices and even present-day acupuncturists will use Quartz-tipped needles. If you have ever sung into a microphone or laid a needle down on a vinyl record spinning on a gramophone, you have listened to the sound of crystal energy reverberating energy back to you through the sound of music or your voice.

The first microphones and gramophone needles were made with pieces of quartz because of their piezoelectric qualities. This means that Quartz has the ability to change energy from one form to another. You can even measure a change in its shape when you conduct electricity or voltage through it. Not many people understand that Quartz is an electrical conduit and should be studied more deeply and heavily for these purposes. It has all too often been discounted as just another New Age bobble that people like to put on their dashboards and next to their bedside tables to get a better night's sleep.

What actually happens when people do that is that the crystal emits an energy frequency that changes the vibration of the space around it. If you fall asleep with a crystal next to your head on your bedside table, then you will change your sleep patterns and perhaps even elicit more interesting dreams as a result.

When you are in contact with an energy frequency that is different from your own you will have a subtle change or shift in your own frequency that can cause either higher or lower vibrational frequency. In the case of the Quartz crystal which emanates a frequency higher than most objects you will encounter on a daily basis, it will bring a higher, more positive frequency toward your energy and give you a little push upward.

It was Nikola Tesla, the Father of Electricity, who said that if we want to understand the Universe, then we need to study and understand the concepts of vibration and frequency. The reality of these two energetic components is that they describe through pulsation and light that they are coming from a certain dynamic life-force or quality of existence. It is like reading a map of someone's body, or a map of a continent you have never visited.

The energy frequency of all things is the imprint or signature of that object, being, or place. Even some places on Earth have stronger or higher vibrational frequencies and are sometimes referred to as vortexes. In these locations, people have reported feeling the sudden onset of vertigo, nausea, or a feeling of being high, just from standing in these spots. Not all people are ready to experience such a shift in energy and that is why there can be an unpleasant feeling at first. In general, however, these sensations are vibrational frequencies that are allowing us to feel how powerful and strong that energy is.

What happens when you try and push two, opposing magnets together? About a ¼ to a ½ inch away from each other, they push each other apart. The distance between them is dependent on the quality of the quantum energy of the magnet. These two magnets, when flipped around, will draw each other together so quickly, you better hope your fingers aren't in the way. They each have a positive and negative charge and will quickly decide what they are wanting to touch or be attracted to.

Energy works in these terms and the vibrational frequencies of a magnet are such that it allows them to have such a strong force in both opposing and positive directions. Quartz and other crystals have an energetic imprint just as a magnet does, though many of them are not magnetic themselves. They have other properties, qualities, and characteristics that provide a certain sensation, feeling attitude, or energy that will help you alter your state of being just by holding it in your hand.

Next time you hold a crystal in your hand, ask yourself what it feels like. Our general tendencies are to notice how it looks and to find all of its excitement in the color, shape, and size, but what about the frequency?

Did you know that a lot of people will feel drawn to certain crystal and gemstones on purpose? A lot of us aren't even noticing when we are in a connection to another energy and are being pulled toward it. You could say this about a romantic partnership and the energy of meeting someone new and falling in love. There is a magnetic pull and attraction to the other because your frequencies are in a closer balance to each other, among other things.

With crystals, it won't be quite as romantic, but a similar principle applies.

The energy inside of you is drawn to whatever healing stone you are in need of, in many instances. This is not always the case, and sometimes it takes a lot of practice to get to a mindset where you can actually let yourself be pulled toward what you need. Crystal energy is pulling and repelling energy in ways like a magnet with opposing sides might.

Your energy is a reflection of what you need or what you already have, so if you are drawn to a piece of lapis lazuli on sight and then hold it in your hand and feel a vibrational charge in the palm of your hand, you may be in need of what that stone is offering in the form of frequency. In this case, lapis lazuli resonates with the frequency of the throat chakra and is helpful in opening your self-expression, creativity, and healing the wounds of your inner voice and truth.

Chapter 5: Meanings Of Healing Gemstones

Since ancient civilizations humans have been making use of the energy that is generated by crystals to release blockages that are mental, physical, and even emotional, enabling the energy present in the body to flow freely. Both the cellular structure of the human body and that of a quartz crystal are made of mineral silicone dioxide. Accordingly, human bodies tend to naturally open to the energy transmitted by these crystals. These crystals store energy within themselves.

When such energized crystals are placed in direct contact with your body, such an action will have an extremely powerful effect because of the power transmitted to you from them. One of the popular laws of physics states that thoughts are capable of directing the flow of energy and therefore energy follows thoughts. Each crystal helps us connect to our body on a conscious level. Let's examine the different types of crystals.

Abalone is a gorgeous shell of the ocean, and is thought to possess energy that is both therapeutic and naturally comforting. The multidimensional, muted rainbow colors improve compassionate feelings of love, beauty, and harmony. It was considered to be a revered shell by Native Americans and they used to combine it with sage, in order to communicate their messages to heaven. Abalone is admirable to wear when you need direction, especially in regards to a relationship.

Agate is considered to be amongst one of the most ancient of stones used for the purpose of healing. Agate is believed to be a stone of power and, accordingly, many of the ancient civilizations around the world made use of this in their weapons and armors; in order that it would bring them triumph in the battlefield. It is a shielding stone that is ideal for making amulets. Agates not only bring power but also carry courage, strength, and self-confidence to the wearer.

Amethyst, according to popular belief, is supposed to help in relieving stress and increase one's inner strength, together with bringing a clear sense of commerce to the wearer of this stone. This stone is considered to be a protective shield and aids in bringing prosperity to the person carrying it. Amethyst also aids in cleansing one's mind of all unnecessary thoughts and facilitates in reconnecting with your feelings, allowing to gain a deeper understanding of yourself. These crystals are capable of warding of negative energy and draw out positive energy. These properties of Amethyst make it an excellent choice of protective stone for your home, because they get rid of unnecessary, negative energy.

Aquamarine helps in cleansing the mind and also helps in balancing emotions and strengthening inner powers. Sailors used to carry this stone to defend themselves against the likely perils they would face on their voyage and to increase their strength. Aquamarine is believed to vibrate at a frequency that is similar to that of the heart chakra. Thus, this crystal will help you realize your true self and also form a stronger bond with yourself.

Aventurine is believed by many to be one of the most popular stones, and is thought to bring its wearer luck and blessing the wearer with abundance and success. This stone has the capacity to protect and harmonize the energy radiated by the heart and it also provides with the little push required when it comes to love. This stone facilitates the process of manifestation of one's dreams into reality.

Azurite is considered by many to be a stone of heaven because it helps one in the process of connecting with their spiritual side. This stone is believed to have the energy that can be used to get your spiritual abilities out of their state of inactivity. It is thought to reduce the presence of any unnecessary thoughts, clearing your mind.

Black Tourmalinated Quartz is a type of clear quartz that has got minor fragments of Black Tourmaline embedded within it. Many consider this stone to bring its wearer good luck and health. This stone is believed to help you in release pent up and dormant energy in your body. It also helps remove impediments to energy and neutralize imbalances.

Bloodstone is believed to have therapeutic properties and has been held in great reverence because of its healing functions. All the negative energy present in the body can be removed by means of this crystal, creating greater capacity for positive energy. Bloodstone aids in increasing the core strength of a person and facilitates effortless movements. This is a stone that can be of great use to athletes or any other individual who is engaged in a profession that involves rigorous physical activity.

Blue lace agate is a stone that is capable of removing any blockages that are plaguing the throat chakra. It not only helps you to accept your emotions but it also helps in improving your verbal and communication skills. This stone is considered to be of exceptional use because it can bring its wearer a sense of calm and peace.

Carnelian is a potent sacral chakra stone that improves personal control and physical energy. It provides energy to make you more compassionate and creative. It helps brings out the creative talents possessed by an individual and aids in the expression of one's true self.

Chrysocolla is considered to have a calming and soothing energy on those who are especially prone to anxiety. The negative energies generated during any hardships or times of transition are diminished by this stone. It is an ideal stone that can be worn 0n a daily basis because of its supporting and soothing properties. It also helps in freeing the hurdles faced by the throat chakra, which balances your emotions. When your emotions are balanced thoroughly, your ability to love also improves.

Chrysoparse is a crystal that has the energy to not just open but also truly awaken your heart chakra, and this provides a potent burst of positive energy to your heart. Thus, this stone helps you to love others unconditionally from your heart. This crystal is believed to be a stone of elegance and understanding; it can promote the positive feelings of joy and contentment within a person. This stone also helps elevate the perception of you and removes any undesirable feelings of inadequacy or even superiority.

Citrine is perceived by many to be a stone of happiness and light. It does not hold even an inkling of negative energy and therefore you don't have to cleanse this stone. This stone brings simplicity to the wearer and helps you transform your dreams into reality. Citrine helps in clearing your cluttered thoughts and frees the mind of any negative energy. This stone helps in revitalizing the body and mind.

Clear quartz is a stone that is used to manifest the energy required to unlock all the energy centers that are present within the body. It helps in removing any unnecessary thoughts and brings clarity to the wearer. The clearance of those thoughts allows the wearer to realize their dreams and see what they need to do to achieve their dreams. It helps ensure that there are no obstacles to the flow of energy in the body so that spiritual growth of an individual can unfold.

Coral has often been referred to as the garden of the sea and is considered to have the ability to ward of ill fortune and to provide protection from various skin diseases. When an individual dreams of corals, it is considered to be a good omen that signifies the recovery from a long-suffering ailment. Coral is the color of our life force: blood and is therefore a good crystal to use while meditating.

Fresh water pearls are those pearls that have been cultured in inland waters instead of the ocean. The earliest record of a pearl worn was by a Persian queen in 4300 BC. These pearls are thought to usher in love and magnificence. They also aid you in becoming aware of not just your problems but also of those around you. Pearls are generally associated with purity and help us in experiencing life by being empathetic towards others.

Garnet is considered to be a stone that is associated with both health and power. It is said to possess the energy that is capable of increasing passion and happiness. Garnet facilitates the unobstructed flow of energy within the body and motivates physical activity. This is an ideal stone that one can use to deal with sadness because it brings joy and hope to the person wearing it. It also clears the chakras of any unnecessary energy and revitalizes them.

Goldstone is consists of two elements, copper and quartz glass. The copper embedded within it provides the shimmering look to it. The way the goldstone sparkles is often linked with light that has the power to drive away negative energy. Light can always dispel dark and this stone is used as a protective talisman to ward away negative energies. This leaves the accumulation of positive energies.

Hematite is considered to be a protective stone that has a grounding effect on its wearer. This stone is capable of absorbing negative energy and is extremely helpful to control your anxiety, to stay calm, and remain focused. This will assist you in removing any self-imposed limitations.

Jade is considered to be a powerful talisman and is believed to be able to assist you accomplish your goals. It allows you to see beyond self-imposed boundaries and helps you transform your dreams into reality. Jade encourages courage, empathy, and kindness. This encouragement helps you lead a more affluent and fulfilling life

Labradorite cleanses and helps in awakening the seventh chakra, the crown chakra and facilitates in motivating the wearer's insight. It is considered to be an extremely powerful stone that can help you transform your dreams and aspirations into reality with the means of resolve.

Moonstone is considered by many to be the stone that can reveal a person's destiny. Like the name suggests, this stone has a strong affinity towards the moon and also with women. It is an exceptionally useful stone for women. It is worn with the intention to increase a person's fertility and also to align the mind with the body. It facilitates in bringing forth deep-seated feelings to the foreground.

Mother of Pearl is considered to have extremely powerful energy that is good for healing and is believed to have the power to ward off evil and negative energy. Mother of Pearl is thought to protect innocence and bring good luck, bounty, and splendor.

Obsidian is a volcanic glass produced in the nature when the extremely hot molten lava has rapidly cooled down. Obsidian has grounding effects on the wearer and is believed to help in establishing a strong connection with the root chakra. Obsidian helps you get rid of any pessimistic energy and also helps the wearer let go of negative feelings.

Onyx has both influential and protective characteristics. It helps in forming a defense for the body and mind against the electromagnetic. It absorbs and transforms unhelpful energy, facilitating in the prevention of draining of your personal energy. Onyx helps the wearer let go of negative energy, sadness, and gloominess. It also helps to tone down your fears, thereby making you feel more secure and stable.

Pyrite is also known as fool's gold because of its golden color. This is believed to have the energy to help deal with financial crisis and also helps in attracting opulence. Its likeliness to gold makes this stone a symbol for not just good luck but wealth too. This stone is often linked to the sun because of its radiance and is helpful in fortifying the mind. It is a protective stone.

Rhodonite facilitates in the balancing of emotions and calming of impatience. It is a very helpful crystal that removes blockages faced by the heart chakra. It helps in removing any unnecessary energy and attracts love and balance in all the areas of your life. It also helps you to discover your hidden talents so that they can be put to good use.

Rhodochrosite helps in improving your perception of yourself and helps you to love yourself. This is an extremely powerful crystal and is used for emotional healing. It also facilitates in the process of attaining a state of sheer bliss and has an effect on the heart chakra. It also provides you with the courage required to deal with those things that you might have ignored previously due to the fear of failure.

Rose Quartz is believed to be a stone of unconditional love. This is considered to be an extremely significant stone associated with the heart chakra and the energy generated from this stone can help neutralize any imbalances in this chakra. This stone helps remove any unnecessary feelings like jealousy, anger, envy and so on. Rose quartz fosters love and the formation of bonds that aren't based on brittle foundations.

Rudraksha seeds are considered to be miracle seeds and they give out positive energy. According to the ancient scriptures, Vedas, Rudraksha seeds were created from the tears shed by Lord Shiva for humanity, and therefore these seeds have been sent by the divinity to help humanity heal. These seeds are of extreme spiritual significance and have been worn by sages since the Vedic times.

Rutilated quartz is a type of clear quartz that has fine needle like structures of golden rutile embedded within it. Imbalances and blockages of all the chakras can be removed by making use of this stone. This helps in the process of harmonizing the body and mind to facilitate in the development of an individual. This stone is considered to have the ability to inspire the feelings of joy and happiness in the wearer. Rutilated quartz is also believed to enable the process of faster healing of injuries and to slow down of aging process.

Selenite is the go to crystal for all types of clearing of energies. This stone has the power to not just clear but also protect the energy present in an individual. All the dormant energy that has become stagnant can be removed by making use of this crystal. This crystal can be used for charging other crystals too; you simply need to place the other crystals on it to revitalize them. This crystal has also found to be of use in holistic treatments of various ailments.

Serpentine is a crystal that is believed to possess the powers to reduce any hormonal imbalances and restore balance. If at all there are any blockades present in the chakra this stone can help in removing them so that the process of healing of chakras can be carried on. It helps you to understand that your life can be what you desire it to be and that you are solely responsible for it. This stone often serves the purpose of reminding the wearer that everything is possible and only you have the power to achieve what you want. Thus it is used to achieve all the things you want in life.

Smoky quartz is said to be a stone that can make you one with the Earth. It is believed to have the ability to keep you firmly grounded and lets you be impartial. The energy generated by this stone eliminates any negative energy that is present within you. This stone also helps in doing away with any emotional and mental blocks presents to diminish the presence of negative energy. It helps to reduce negative feelings such as anger, pain, and bitterness.

Sodalite encourages being true to yourself and making a stand for the things you believe in. This stone represents and promotes self-expression and confidence required to deal with any situation. This stone helps in making you believe in your own decisions and also has the ability to facilitate in the development of one's true self.

Sunstone is of great use because of the powerful bond it has with the sun and the energy emanated by the sun. This stone is said to have the power to bring an inkling of positive light to any situation. Thus, it promotes a positive and cheerful attitude. The energy generated by this stone can dispel any dark mood and encourages positive stimuli.

Tiger's Eye is a crystal that is considered to have the energy to restore the balance to your body on different levels and is helpful in restoring one's confidence and faith in the future. The brilliant energy emanated by this stone is believed to bring luck and prosperity to the individual wearing it and because of this reason, it has been used as a talisman by many ancient civilizations.

Turquoise is a beautiful blue green stone that is considered to have special healing properties. This stone is supposed to be the bridge that links heaven and earth. The body can be connected with the Cosmos by making use of this stone, and many of the Native American Tribes believe this. Not only the Native Americans, but also the Chinese healers have special regard for turquoise. This stone is often associated with the throat chakra and is believed to help in leveling any imbalances present in this chakra.

This provides the foundation for all that you will need to know about the different types of crystals that can be made use of in the process of healing one's body, mind, and soul. Each crystal serves a different purpose. Accordingly, depending upon the requirement of the situation, one must use the appropriate crystals.

Chapter 6: Clean And Charge Crystals With The Power Of Earth, Air, Fire, And Water

Precious stones can mystically improve and enable every piece of your life. Everything from straightforward relaxation procedures to mending medical issues or notwithstanding finding past experiences! When you discover a gem or when a precious stone discovers you, the principal thing you need to do is purify and charge your treasure. There are numerous approaches to do this. Here are a couple of choices for you, recorded underneath the vital sign they relate with.

WATER Natural water: Sea, stream, cascade, waterway. Hold the precious stone in the water and let it wash over it. A few precious stones can wind up frail and harmed by water, for example, powder.

Saltwater: Equal parts cold water and ocean salt. A few gems can't be placed legitimately in seawater (like opals). It might harm the structure of the precious stone, change the completion, or change the shade of the gem. You can likewise put the precious stone in a little bowl of water at that point place that bowls into a bowl of salt, so the salt encompasses the gem without direct contact with the salt.

EARTH You can cover your precious stone in a nursery or pruned the plant and leave for 24 hrs. When you include it in a greenhouse, make sure you mark the spot so you can discover it once more, and furthermore make sure any pets you have won't uncover it.

Gem Cluster: Place your precious stone on a "piece" or "bunch" of clear quartz or amethyst medium-term. You can likewise utilize a little glass bowl of tumbled hematite stones. Additionally, leave medium-term.

Rice: Place precious stone in a little glass bowl with uncooked natural rice. Cover the precious stone in the rice for 24 hrs. At that point, dispose of the rice when you did.

FIRE Candle fire: Hold precious stone and rapidly go it through the candle fire or you can encompass your gem with tea light candles and leave consuming till they all wear out.

AIR Incense: Light incense (attempt wise or lavender). Hold precious stone and run it through the smoke. Utilize your hand or a plume to direct smoke towards and through the precious stone.

Smearing: Same as incense, light smudge stick and victory, run your gem through the smoke. Utilize your hand or plume too. Sage is likewise prescribed.

When you have cleaned your gem from every single negative vitality, you have to charge your precious stone. To do that you mainly grasp the precious stone while imaging all the negative energy leaving the gem, see a dull fog glide away or disintegrate away, at that point fill the flower with brilliant white light. See it filling the whole precious stone and envision it transmitting with only unadulterated positive vitality. See the precious stone in your "mind's eye" as clean, clear, and positively charged. Presently your precious stone is a great idea to proceed to prepared for use.

There are numerous approaches to utilize precious stones to improve and enable your life. You can wear them, as in adornments, and I'm not discussing the costly precious stones and rubies. You can discover delightful precious stones for by nothing and can even make your adornments if you're the imaginative kind. You can convey gems with you in a pocket or handbag for individual protection, place them around your home to lift pessimism and keep up a cheerful home. You can think with them, fortune tells with them and even analyze and mend your very own medical issues with precious stones. Precious stones can do astounding things, and if you let them, they can always change your life!

Are our precious stones new to you? It is safe to say that you are searching for various and intriguing approaches to clean or charge your precious stones? Open the intensity of the four components! You can clean your precious stones by utilizing the earth, air, water, and fire! Okay, prefer to have the option to identify and mend your medical issues? Are you ever needed to know your identity in your past life? Need to go on a thoughtful voyage into the very center of the gem? Start your experience with the intensity of earth, air, water, and fire and let it change your life for eternity.

How to Use a Crystal Ball

Stage 1. Planning

A great many people discover precious stone ball looking is most straightforward in a calm, faintly lit room. Numerous individuals like to have candles consuming. For some the impressions of the flares help to gather images - others discover them a diversion. Consuming incense is standard, and a few people like to have calming music playing tenderly in the background. The significant thing to recollect is that you are making a climate.

The significant key when doing precious stone ball looking is that you should be loose, and your mind must be clear. It is always best to play out a purifying custom pursued by an assurance custom and afterward, start your precious stone ball work. Ordinarily, a purifying tradition would be performed on night one. The following night you would play out a security custom on yourself, and inside the room, you plan on playing out the precious stone ball looking. On the third night, you would then be able to be solid and steady to utilize your expensive stone ball. Even though these customs do not need, it is always savvy to do them for most extreme wellbeing and best outcomes.

When playing out any scrying or divination, you are bringing forth powers from the soul domain. Typically these powers are deterred from this plane we live in except if otherwise aggravated, for example, through clear customs, for example, precious stone ball looking and scrying. When you perform divination, these powers can either help you in delivering images of things to come or different occasions or assault you.

Insidiousness spirits and negative impacts can utilize your precious stone ball, scrying mirror, ouija board, or pendulum a connection for them to venture through into this world. They can likewise use it as a way to empty vitality of you too. This is the reason it is always best to guarantee appropriate purifying, and assurance is set up beforehand.

Stage 2. The Crystal Ball Gazing Method

Spot the gem ball on a table before you. Numerous precious stone balls you can purchase accompany their very own stand. If you don't have an expensive stone ball stand you may get a kick out of the chance to utilize a little pad or a silk tissue bought and saved extraordinarily for this reason.

Tip

To intensify your precious stone ball looking, you can utilize a gemstone circle as a compliment to the gem ball. Mostly having a gemstone circle resting next the expensive stone ball can enlarge your plunging two creases.

Plunk down and unwind. Lay your hands tenderly on the ball for a moment or two to empower it and reinforce your mystic affinity. While holding the precious stone ball, consider the reason for this scrying session if the proper attempt to envision the subject of your inquiry. A few people like to pose the investigation for all to hear; others want to disguise it.

Presently, expel your hands from the precious stone. Investigate the precious stone, gaze profoundly. Enable your eyes to unwind and turn out to be somewhat unfocused. After a short time, you should see a fog or smoke framing in the gem. Allow this to fog develop and fill the ball, at that point imagine it bit by bit clearing to uncover images inside the precious stone.

The images you see probably won't be what you anticipated. That is OK, don't battle them. Your intuitive personality realizes what data you need. Numerous individuals find that when they initially start to utilize a gem ball, the images have nothing to do with what they center around. This is because your psyche isn't yet balanced at having the option to handle and concentrate on the energies being passed from your intuitive into the gem ball itself. Think about the psychological strengths going from your brain to the gym ball as a pipe. The base or "tip" of the channel is your subliminal energies, and that vitality is being coordinated upwards towards your conscious personality, which is the mid purpose of the pipe. The informed piece of the mind that gets the subliminal energy then "spills" it into the gem ball to frame those images from the psyche, which would be the mouth of the pipe.

Since divination utilizes both the subconscious and informed piece of the brain simultaneously, it very well may be reasonably hard to focus on both without a moment's delay. Your subliminal is the place the vitality is coming from. It passes it upwards to your cognizant which is expected to follow up on that vitality into the gem ball. Without the conscious personality, you would be in all the more a profound ruminated state and your eyes would not have the option to intentionally center or info the images inside the precious stone ball.

As noted, it is flawlessly OK that the first couple times you divine with a gem ball the images are not identified with what it is you need. The reality you can see ANYTHING in the precious stone ball is indicating progress. The more you work with the expensive stone ball, the better you will get at having the option to see precisely what it is you need to see by controlling your intuitive energies to your cognizant strengths, and after that to the gem ball. In any case, let the images stream, changing, and taking you any place they go. Try not to attempt to legitimize currently, time for that later.

Stage 3. Shutting The Crystal Ball Session

Let the images gradually blur over into the gem ball. Don't merely stop the session all of a sudden, slightly invert the procedure you utilized toward the start. Envision the fogs returning and covering the images, at that point retreating to restore the ball to its normal state.

Thank you for the precious stone ball and put it away painstakingly wrapped inside a dim material is best as dark fabric keeps the energies of the ball contained inside it and keeps it from spilling out.

It is likewise always best to guarantee you rinse your precious stone ball. A decent, quick, and primary way of doing this is to light a savvy smirch stick as well as wise incense and move the ball around the smoke before you place it back for capacity. Another quick and simple way to scrub your precious stone ball is to give it a dunk in salt water for about one moment. You would prefer not to douse it excessively long in salt as it can harm and destroy the precious stone ball.

Distance Crystal Healing

Separation Crystal Healing (DCH) is one of the best mending treatments accessible on earth today. There is, anyway, some vital data that you should know before you take an interest in Crystal Healing (CH). Whenever done effectively, separation precious stone recuperating can transform you.

Gem Healing

Any sort of recuperating finished with precious stones can be incredibly unusual and should be taken care of with deference and consideration. The very characteristics of precious stone, as a guide to alternative prescription, make gem a perfect course for alternative treatments. Precious stone has been utilized for quite a long time as a demonstrated scientific strategy for intensifying vitality. Health and wellbeing can likewise be increased in your vitality field by securely using the expanded amplification of the recuperating treatment.

CH treatment is very flexible and is done in numerous comprehensive health structures. For instance, some basic alternative health strategies that use precious stones are gem recuperating music, reiki, stones, gem wands, singing dishes, vitality mending gem, pranic mending, vibrational medication, quantum separation mending, chakra adjusting, contemplation ... furthermore, the rundown continues forever. CH keeps on being found for its numerous outstanding health benefits.

Separation Healing

Separation recuperating is an astounding type of moving vitality and expanding health. Mental, enthusiastic, and physical health would all be able to be improved by the correct treatment run using separation. It is tough for specific individuals to see how incredible a long divorce recuperating can be. As a matter of fact, with the right preparing, a health professional can figure out how to convey a recuperating treatment by separation session, that makes better outcomes, than if the customer was in the room. Usually, the comprehensive specialist must be an abnormal state recuperating supplier and prepared in specific alternative mending treatments.

Separation Healing rises above the limits of existence, permitting people to claim intrinsic dismantle towards equalization to stream uninhibitedly. The centralization of nurturing vitality sent to the customer is more grounded when done through the long separation channel. Mending influences can be substantially more immediate.

Separation Crystal Healing

It is obvious to see that when you put the amplified mending forces of precious stone together with the immediate laser-likely focal point of separation recuperating ... you have joined the best of two universes. DCH can have significant health benefits. Health upgrades can be picked up in a wide range of zones, and issues of any nature can be reduced. Physical, mental, and intense subject matters can discover alleviation with the protected and appropriate utilization of these alternative remedial techniques.

Crystal Healing - Do Crystal and Gemstone Healing Therapies Work?

Gems and gemstones have been esteemed for quite a long time for their excellence and furthermore for their recuperating powers. It is accepted that the antiquated Egyptians were propelled, gem healers.

There is the way of thinking that exists that these Egyptian healers may have gotten their propelled learning in the utilization of gems in the recuperating expressions from their antecedents, the general population of Atlantis.

They realized that through the incitement of unobtrusive vibrational frequencies in the human vitality field, or air, recuperating could happen in people and creatures. At the point when specific stones were put on the body in critical territories and permitted to stay there for a brief timeframe, the individual getting the treatment improved.

Cutting edge acupuncturists comprehend this idea and use needle therapy needles to animate a portion of the extremely same zones that the Egyptian healers used to put their mending stones.

By setting precious stones and gemstones in the closeness of specific chakras, meridians, and another vitality focuses, blockages become cleared and recuperating is encouraged.

Individuals regularly experience a sentiment of shivering or vibration in the territories that the precious stones and gemstones are put on their body during a gem recuperating session.

Old recollections and fears may flood into their psyches immediately, and afterward, all of a sudden be discharged. A few people feel torments facilitating, muscles unwinding, firmness of joints and bones easing, and sentiment of harmony, tranquility, and clearness tenderly beating them.

During a precious stone recuperating session it isn't bizarre for an individual getting a treatment to re-experience an old injury, as though its stifled memory has re-surfaced as it is leaving the air or vitality field, and the physical body at the same time.

At the point when an individual discharge an old, blocked passionate or physical damage along these lines, they get an opportunity to see the past circumstance through unexpected eyes in comparison to when they initially experienced it. Maybe they are more established now or have become more shrewd, so now they can at long last look at what occurred before, and ideally have the vital instruments to process that old injury, and let it go for good.

It is astonishing how much physical torment can be attached to old passionate damages. By discharging them and releasing them along these lines, a few people find that they have another rent on life.

Since this sort of treatment is viewed as careless, an individual may languish with an issue over numerous prior years, figuring out how to effectively manage it.

Directing and mental treatment has frequently been the primary alternative for specific individuals, and it can at times take a long time to work through an issue that may be discharged through an evening with a decent gem recuperating expert.

Gems and gemstones can be utilized to adjust the vitality bodies, carrying parity to the physical, passionate, mental, and the profound existences of people. This enables individuals to discover alleviation from long-standing afflictions rather rapidly where other customary medications have been fruitless.

This sort of treatment is something that must be experienced to be accepted. Similarly, as with anything strange, you will consistently have cynics who question the legitimacy of this sort of recuperating methodology.

In any case, When you have been experiencing something that you have been ineffective in treating, you may need to genuinely think about this unwinding, non-intrusive, safe elective treatment.

Crystal Healing: Is It a Myth or Does It Work?

Ancient Indian culture and numerous societies in the East accept that stones do have amending power. The human body has seven chakras; the vitality focuses that are situated in the midline of the body beginning from the base of the spine till the crown. When it is contrasted with the life systems of the body, every chakra is related to an endocrine organ. Vitality must stream uninhibitedly through each of the chakras, which guarantees good health, significant serenity, and concordance. So also, appropriate working of every endocrine organ ensures physical and psychological wellness. Shading and stone represent each chakra. These stones are known as the chakra mending stones. The vitality of the stones unblocks the chakras and parities the energy for good health and prosperity.

Present-day science has continuously dismissed the case that gem mending truly works. With the utilization of gems, the chakras (endocrine) capacities can be recuperated. An ongoing report has demonstrated that the subjects experienced some glow, shivering sensation, and sentiment of prosperity or abhorrence when in contact with stones.

Gem healers and recuperating specialists have built up a top to bottom information of the stones, mineral, and gems, which are utilized as back rub stones, precious stone treatment stones or mending stones. Spa culture has advanced, where the advisor offers back rubs using spa stones. Regardless of whether a devotee or not, the utilization of rocks for a back rub or mending or just embellishment has a constructive outcome of the psyche on the individual as they have various types and levels of energies.

Is precious stone mending a legend?

The volunteers were prepared concerning what's in store and what they can understanding. Some were given phony gemstones, while some were given genuine ones. All subjects experienced what they were advised to anticipate. This implies the human personality can be prepared and molded to plan a specific arrangement of results or sensations as the result of the trial/test.

How does recuperating precious stones work?

Our whole body is a vitality that is communicated in various examples and densities. At the point when all the spirit works in an amicable case, the intelligent life alludes to good health. Any unsettling influence or unevenness in the liver causes malady and sick health, which might be physical, mental, or passionate.

All stones are known to have energies. The gemstones radiate vitality in a specific example, at a wavelength because of the arrangement of the subatomic particles. Gem healers and specialists comprehend the case that resounds in our body and supplements it with the example radiated by the gem treatment stones. An offset is made with the standards which help the body to unblock the chakras and license-free progression of vitality.

Mending is fundamentally recuperation; utilization of recuperating stones is an all-encompassing way to deal with good health. With no known reactions, the utilization of precious stone recuperating stones is a useful method to recover good health, significant serenity, and satisfaction.

What is Crystal Healing?

Our present comprehension of material science teaches us that all issue in presence is comprised of vitality. Light is composed of specific wavelengths, and everything with mass is composed of little particles, which incorporates the human body and the energy that courses through it.

Each sort of molecule that exists has a specific recurrence on which it vibrates. This is something that antiquated holistic medication shares practically speaking with present-day science lessons; no piece of the human body is ever still.

Specialists in precious stone recuperating keep up the conviction that particular kinds of diseases come about because of awkward nature in the body that have happened. They have learned throughout the years that there is nothing extraordinary about the vibrational recurrence of the issue in the human body, and in that, there are likewise numerous components that can be found in nature that offer these vibrational examples.

Various kinds of precious stone, for instance, are said by advocates of gem mending to have indistinguishable lively properties from crucial individual vitality focuses on the body.

Similarly that setting distinctive sound speakers together that are playing something very similar can cause an expansion in the volume of the sound through amicable wave intensification, putting a particular kind of precious stone that offers the recurrence of vibration that a specific piece of the body does that might experience the ill effects of a type of ailment can improve the natural waves of that territory.

Precious stones, in this sense, go about as a directing reference point to improve the progression of natural energies through pieces of the body that might encounter shortcoming, and after some time this gem was mending and help to reestablish physical quality.

Individuals who have undergone this kind of holistic treatment have revealed odd sensations after investing some energy with the exceptional mending precious stones in contact with their bodies. It's nearly just as they're suddenly mindful of their heartbeat, yet only in the zone that the stone is physically contacting. This is very abnormal since we are generally incapable of feeling our beating beat independent from anyone else.

Specialists in the field of gem mending would state this is the sentiment of flow that is upgrading and improving at a rate that the body isn't utilized to. It's a decent sign that the people natural vibrational energies are being reestablished to a healthy state.

Mending by methods for gems can likewise profoundly affect the patient's psychological state. Mental blockages can be significantly more hard to analyze than physical ones since they don't always show themselves in a manner that is promptly evident to somebody that isn't touchy to them.

In any case, precious stone mending can give away to patients to come into a condition of recharged mental clarity, and a short time later they may have a simpler time getting rid of negative behavior patterns that cost them previously.

The Facts About Crystal Healing

Precious stones have been utilized to reestablish harmony and fix afflictions since the seasons of old Egypt. The conviction is that negative vitality is discharged and cleared through their utilization. By freeing ourselves of negative energies, we help our bodies in recuperating.

Notwithstanding records demonstrating the utilization of precious stones in old Egypt records likewise go back 5,000 years showing their use in Ayurvedic and conventional Chinese drug rehearses too. Recuperating with gems utilizes the use of gemstones for mending repeats.

The stones are put on "chakras" or vitality focuses of the body. It is thought to reinforce the body by settling infirmities with different kinds of gems which convey various rates of vibration. Because of the changing mineral content accessible in each sort of flower, everyone will give its one of a kind vibration. Precious stones can be utilized for mending physical, enthusiastic, mental, and profound lopsided characteristics.

To utilize precious stones for recuperating, one can wear them as an adornment, place them around the tub while they wash or keep them close to their bed while snoozing.

Following are the absolute most regular kinds of gems and a clarification of their recuperating properties.

Clear Quartz - Assists the body in reestablishing wellbeing by unblocking vitality focuses. One can improve their resistant framework by holding a quartz point each day. This kind of gemstone will dispose of negative energies and work to center the brain.

Rose Quartz - Its delicate pink tone is calming. It can help dauntlessness of confidence when it is being tried. It is a quieting stone that identifies with self-esteem. It causes one to discharge outrage and different sentiments of pessimism by empowering forgiveness.

Smokey Quartz - This is a good karma precious stone. It was utilized amid the fight when old troopers expected to advance unwinding and hose pessimism.

Its most normal use is to put it under the pad while you are dozing. It is said to initiate bright dreams. It causes one to review exercises and parity of sexual vitality.

Amethyst - This stone is lilac or profound purple in shading. It is characteristic of innovativeness and one's capacity to rehearse otherworldly recuperating. It can decrease bad dreams when held under one's pad and can improve REM rest. It is now and again used to mend liquor addiction.

Citrine - This stone is beautiful yellow or deep orange in shading. Precious stone mending happens when one is encountering pressure and tension when one holds it close by. It is additionally said to help one in the improvement of relational abilities.

Chapter 7: Crystsl Shapes

These exclusive crystals often look like rods or wands, however they are unique because they have points on both ends. These crystals are very powerful because they have the ability to transmit and emit energy from two places. Sometimes one end may be releasing energy while the other point is transmitting energy, other times both points may be transmitting or emitting energy. Because of this, they have many purposes, but should be used with care.

The Massage Wand:

Perfect for massage therapists, this type of crystal has no pointed end at all, but rather two rounded ends, with one end being wider than the opposite. They are popular amongst massage therapists and reflexologists.

The Double Pointed Crystal:

These unique crystals often look like rods or wands, however they are unique because they have points on both ends. These crystals are very powerful because they have the ability to transmit and emit energy from two places. Sometimes one end may be releasing energy while the other point is transmitting energy, other times both points may be transmitting or emitting energy. Because of this, they have many purposes, but should be used with care.

The Laser Wand:

This crystal is characteristically clear in color, is long in length, but narrows at the tip. This kind of crystal is popular amongst energy workers and acupuncturists. This crystal is very powerful, and concentrates all of its energy around the tip. Only use this crystal with positive, direct intentions.

The Pendulum:

This prevalent crystal shape can easily be made into a necklace or used as a pendulum. When worn, this crystal is a great protector and healer. It also identifies imbalances in the human body. As a pendulum, this crystal can be used for a wide array of purposes, mainly by experienced energy workers.

The Sphere:
This rounded crystal is always manmade, but that is because the sphere is a powerful shape, making these crystals extremely powerful. The sphere crystal emits energy in all directions equally and is helpful when meditating, as well as trying to connect with your innermost self.

The Cube:
Numerous crystals come in the shape of a cube. This shape is able to harvest a significant amount of energy and can be very stabilizing. Like the calculated nature of their shape, these crystals are easy to program and are known to secure intentions well.

The Egg:
This exact kind of crystal is known for its aesthetic beauty. These types of crystals are popular among those who practice acupressure as well as reflexologists. Egg shaped crystals are known for holding energy that can find an imbalance within the body.

The Heart:

The heart shaped crystal is known to attract loving energy, as well as energies that can help those with negative emotions. This healing crystal deals with the mental body, and works to deter sadness, grief, suffering and pain. The heart crystal has also been known to increase fertility.

Sacred Geometry Shapes:

Some crystals may resemble one of the sacred geometry shapes. These crystals are highly spiritual and represent all that life is composed of, giving them the name "platonic solids". These crystals are very useful for aligning the chakras and during meditation.

The Tower:

This crystal is fairly even on all sides and is aerodynamic, designed to stand up on its own. The best tower shaped crystals are formed so that a pointed tip is at the top of the tower, almost like a castle. These crystals are very powerful and can energize anything that comes near it. Use these tower crystals with caution.

The Pencil:

This crystal is long, narrow, and features one pointed end and one dull end. It looks quite like a pencil, hence the name. They are used by experienced energy workers looking to create a crystal grid, and by casual crystal healers for everyday use.

The Pointed Crystal:

This is one of the most common shapes of crystals, and it features one pointed end and one rugged end. This crystal can be used for a wide array of healing practices, and is a good shape for beginners. Most often, clear quartz is found in this shape.

The Wand:

This long crystal has one rounded end, one pointed end, and is typically wider on the round side. Wands are usually manmade, but are great healing crystals because it is easy to direct the flow of energy with them.

Crystal grid

Making a crystal grid
- Example of Crystal grid

Mostly used to amplify the vibration energy of a crystal, grids made of healing stones can help you through the toughest of times without a scratch. Crystal Grids are highly programmed crystal energy mostly used for realizing dreams to healing magic.

Key characteristics that define a Crystal Grid are its trademark. The stones in a crystal grid are divided into various parts for a clearer understanding of crystal physics. Depending on the color and lattice of the grid, these stones are chosen.

Focus stones

Used as a center stone, focus stones should be the most powerful stone with energies that you desire to work on realizing your goal. Technically, Focus Stone multiplies the universal life force to create an energy flow directed downwards.

Way stones

From the center of your crystal grid, the circles of stones around focus stone are the way stones. These stones constitute the most important part of energy flow. Simply put, way stones regulate the flow of energy and chakra through your crystal grid.

Desire Stones

The exterior circle around the focus stone is also third from the center. When appropriately matched, desire stones give body to your goals and desires to make it a reality.

Path

Shortly put as the road to the completion of our desire, the path is the means to your goal. A path is weaved when the crystal grid begins to experience energy transfer in shapes such as circle, square, triangle, quadrilateral, Seeds of a flower, Spirals, Pentagons, Mandalas and Eye of Horus.

Visual

Commanded by color shapes and designs, visual prowess of a crystal grid decides the psychic aura of your grid. For example, if you're asking for rain your crystal grid having a blue ocean like background will amplify your focus.

Benefits of making a crystal grid

Crystal grids are used to double or maximize your power with the use of multiple crystals arranged in a systematic and scientific pattern.

It can help in making you more powerful in addition to making your dreams come true easier than usual.

Crystal grids are highly useful for medicinal purposes as it contains the Universal Life Force capable of life and death.

Things needed to make a crystal grid?

Crystals to cast your wishes right

Crystal Grid made out a chart

Paper with your intentional scenery in the backdrop.

A Sacred Place to practice your crystal power

Quartz crystal to amplify your crystal power

Cleaning incense flavors.

Soft Cloth to dry your crystal

Paper with a list of your goals.

Based on the Color Energies, each crystal can assist differently.

Orange color

An important part of every crystal grid, orange crystals such as Citrine are powerful to enlighten and connect you with the spiritual realm. A crystal to boost your spiritual awareness, use this Citrine for new beginnings as well as protection from psychic attacks.

Green color

Used for the growth of wealth and wisdom, green energy crystals such as jade, when arranged in circles around your central crystal in a grid can attract money or success.

Rose Color

A loving color that fills the wearer with calming vibrations, rose colored crystals such as rose quartz are the epitome of emotional freedom. In fact, rose quartz is an exceptionally powerful crystal with power to let go of leftover love as well as attract your soul mate.

Wear Rose Quartz to find your true love sooner than too late!

Blue color

The color energy of blue is radiant and known to comfort the wearer. Sodalite is ideal for relieving pain due to failures. Use this Sodalite to restore your mental clarity, satisfaction and enthusiasm.

Chapter 8: Crystals For Stress-Relief

How Do I Use Crystals to Relieve Stress?

When your body is experiencing high levels of stress, its natural defenses are weakened, making you more vulnerable to developing physical, mental and emotional illnesses. Thus, stress reduction plays an important role in preserving your wellness and prolonging your life. Simply put, the wisest thing to do would be to use healing crystals before any disease has the chance to manifest.

Stress Reliever Crystal Pattern for the Chakras

Now that you understand where your chakras are located, it should be easy for you to follow this method.

What you'll need:

4 Clear Quartz

3 Amethyst

2 Black Onyx

1 Rose Quartz

Assume a comfortable lying position.

First, lay one amethyst on your third eye chakra. One of the amethysts should be on the palm of your right hand while the other should be held in the palm of your left hand. Its purpose is to ground you and calm you. Furthermore, the positioning of these crystals is essential in guiding the energy up towards your crown chakra then later, back down again to your base chakra.

Next, place one onyx on the sole of your right foot then the other one on the sole of your left foot. The purpose of this is to take away and release the negative energies from your body that are responsible for causing stress.

Place the rose quartz on your abdomen. You need to do this to maintain balance between the female and male energies that all of us possess. Also, place one of the clear quartz on your abdomen, just above the rose quartz.

The second clear quartz should be laid above your head. Place the third beside your arm on the right side. Meanwhile, put the other on the left side. The purpose of these clear quartz crystals is for aura detoxification and chakra cleansing.

When you're done, you would've successfully created dual triangle energy zones with the positioning of the crystals.

Relax your muscles. Close your eyes. Concentrate on your breathing.

Remain in a meditative state for at least 10 minutes or as long as you need.

When it's all over, you may use these crystals as your worry stones. Place them in a silk pouch and bring them with you wherever you go. Each time you feel the familiar symptoms of anxiety creeping in, just reach into your pocket or into your purse, massage the worry stones with your fingers, and draw strength from them.

What can I Do to Lessen Stress and Anxiety at the Workplace?

One of the many purposes of healing crystals is to help you cope with everyday stresses. While it's impossible to completely escape exposure to daily stressors, healing crystals can help minimize their negative effects to your body, your psyche, your emotions and your spirit.

The following stones are highly recommended in reducing stress in the workplace. They also help increase your productivity. More than that, they aid in smoothing your professional relationships.

If you're after career success, then consider owning an **emerald**. This crystal is often used to attract abundance. More importantly, it will help you achieve mental clarity, thus, helping you in figuring out your goals. Keep it on your desk and use it as a visualization tool during brief office breaks.

Some people struggle with establishing healthy professional relationship boundaries. The result is that they get taken advantage of or are treated with less respect than they deserve. In such cases, keeping an **amber** crystal is recommended.

If you're dissatisfied with the circumstances in your workplace and are striving for change, then you may choose to carry an **amethyst** with you. Draw power and courage from it so that you can control a challenging situation at work.

For individuals who are suffering from lack of productivity, a **garnet** is advised. Not only will it boost your energy but also those of your colleagues, team members, or subordinates.

If communication is not your strength, then a **blue lace agate** may prove to be immensely valuable. This will aid you in effectively expressing your ideas with your clients, bosses and co-workers. This crystal is also recommended for individuals who feel like they are looked over, underappreciated and misunderstood.

The **larimar** is another stone, which is effective in clearing pathways of communication. When you find it difficult to understand others, then use this crystal. If you have to work in front of the computer all day long, then consider placing a **purple fluorite** beside it. This way, you'll be protected from the harmful effects of the computer's electromagnetic field.

Is someone taking advantage of you at the office? Is your horrible boss siphoning your soul? Is your toxic workmate pulling you down with him? If such is the case, then carry a **smoky quartz**. This crystal will prevent these emotional vampires from drawing off every last ounce of your energy. If someone in the office is shattering your ego, then this crystal will help increase your self-confidence.

Chapter 9: Bloodstone

The Ancients knew Bloodstone as Heliotrope, a name derived from the two Greek words meaning 'sun-turning' and is said to preserve the mind and body of the wearer and therefore has long been used as a talisman of vibrant health and lasting life. It is a stone known to boost intuition as well as warding off illnesses like colds and flu by invigorating the entire bodily system and may increase overall physical endurance. The bloodstone is a variant of Jasper but in most cases is a mixture of both Jasper and Quartz with dark green hues inset with bright red blood-like spots and flecks. Bloodstone is not just a gemstone worn for its healing properties that include but are certainly not limited to boosting the immune system as well as cleansing and purifying organs such as the bladder, liver, spleen, and intestines, and it is also said that wearing a Bloodstone talisman brings its owner affluence, respect, riches, and even fame. This gemstone of many uses is extraordinary in both appearance and boasts energetic frequencies that offer the user courage and determination and so is the perfect talisman for those suffering in mourning or facing difficult times. This stone holds to both the Root and Heart Chakra and acts to balance and synchronise the body's chakra network and aura by clearing any energetic blockages giving way to levels of heightened understanding which transcend our usual selves. A Bloodstone is often worn by those hoping to make their mark on the earning honour, respect, and prestige.

Colour
Green/Red
Birthstone
March
Zodiac
Aries
Connections to Scorpio
Energetic Frequencies
Acceptance
Magic
Sacrifice
Healing

Chakras
The Heart Chakra
The Root Chakra

Blue John

Found exclusively in Derbyshire England, Blue John displays layers of deep blue, purple, white, reds and yellow. This incredibly popular and charismatic stone is a type of fluorite composition which since Roman times has been used to protect wearers from the effects of drunkenness. This rare stone is popular among collectors with crystals carrying deep purple hues being the most sought after. Blue John's vibrational energy holds many metaphysical properties many of which stem from the powerful calming energy that flood from the stone. It helps to quiet a busy mind, gently breaking destructive and repetitive thought patterns and is renowned for being a catalyst for personal transition, renewal and growth. Wearing Blue John spurs us on to seek out and experience new and exciting things. Meditating with Blue John brings truth and greater understanding into our lives and its connection to the Third Eye Chakra helps to connect us to higher spiritual levels of consciousness and is also known to assist in lucid dreaming. Blue John is a powerful healing stone that works by activating the Crown and Solar Plexus Chakras and is said to assist in healing from infections. Blue John also promotes healthy bone and teeth growth as well as significantly lowering recovery time for broken bones and fractures. It also works well for general pain relief and is great at soothing nerves. Blue John has been used to cure inflammations and irritations of the eyes, ears, nose and throat since Ancient Rome and it has long been known that it stimulates the immune system and the body's natural detoxification processes. This is a stone that works wonders for the mind, improving focus and clarity of thought by drawing in and pooling together our distorted and scattered energies and then realigning them in the way most suited to fulfilling our goals. Blue John's energy supports and encourages us, it helps us to overcome small-mindedness and improper reasoning. It forces us to see truths within ourselves which can be a painful process but serves only to make us stronger in the long run by helping us to discover true meaning. Laying back and placing Blue John on the throat and/or brow is said to allow us access to information and concepts that would otherwise have been utterly inaccessible. Spiritual practitioners commonly use Blue John to enhance clairvoyance and other psychic and it is said that it can even unlock the path to the mystical state of 'No Mind' or 'The Void'.

Colour
Striped bands of:
Blue
Purple
White
Red
Yellow

Birthstone
January
February

Zodiac
Pisces

Energetic Frequencies
Calming
Transformative
Healing
Chakras
The Third Eye Chakra
The Crown Chakra
The Solar Plexus Chakra
Brandberg Amethyst

Brandberg Amethyst is a variation of Smoky Quartz and Amethyst found exclusively in Namibia, specifically the Brandberg (or Fire) Mountain located in the Namib Desert. This is one of the few crystals regularly found with enhydros (inclusions of pure water) and other rare inclusions and imperfections making them valuable to spiritualists, healers, and Reiki practitioners. It is a multi-purpose healing stone that affects us emotionally, spiritually and physically, aligning us with the universal energy that surrounds us and inspiring unconditional love through both thought and action. Brandberg Amethyst combines the calming influence of Amethyst with the grounding effect of

Smokey Quartz culminating in an effect that stabilises the entire bodily system and amplifies and lifts the natural energetic frequency of the chakra network and aura. Brandberg Amethyst is known as a 'master healer' and as such is extremely useful in lowering recovery time from both illness and injury alike. It helps those suffering from chronic fatigue, malnutrition and immune deficiencies through its ability to revitalise the bodily system and realign the natural flow of energy throughout the body and chakra network. The vibrational energy emitted by Brandberg Amethyst when properly harnessed and directed can be used to elevate skeletal and dental pain and is also thought to aid in healing from infections relating to the ears and throat. Brandberg Amethyst has a forceful effect both spiritually and emotionally healing and supporting those suffering from addictions, stress. It is a stone that allows us to let go of past traumas, feelings of guilt, loss and anger, and regret, which ultimately allows us to forgive ourselves and others, providing long-lasting feelings of inner peace and joy. This is a stone that works as a cosmic anchor attaching our energy to that of the earth and one which also has a balancing effect on the chakra network, healing the spirit, revitalising the body and fills the recipient with feelings of contentment and joy.

Colour
Purple
Blue
Opaque
Smokey
Light Yellow/Red
Birthstone
February
November
December
Zodiac
Aquarius
Pisces
Energetic Frequencies
Protection
Healing
Chakras
The Third Eye Chakra
The Crown Chakra

Brochantite

Brochantite is a crystal that exerts a powerful influence over the ethereal body and chakra network of the human body and has been highly prized for its healing properties and ability to realign the body's meridians and all of the chakras. Typically displaying a variation of bright green to dark dull green, Brochantite has also been known to appear with hues of darkest green to black. It is a stone regularly used in meditation practices due to strong connections to the higher spiritual realms, the relaxing effect it has on those who come into contact with its calming energy, and for its purification qualities that turn any space into a safe and relaxing environment in which to meditate or practice healing or prayer. Brochantite is commonly used to realign and centre the chakras. It also has the effect of lifting the vibrational energy of the body bringing out our best selves and bridges the gap between the physical and spiritual realms. The high copper content within Brochantite's makeup makes it a great healing stone and is known to help those plagued by lung and respiratory conditions. It works great for those suffering from water retention, it balances fluids within the bodily system, regulates and maintains a healthy blood flow and has been used in the treatment of illnesses relating to the pancreas and prostate. Brochantite also protects against environmental pollutants and other contaminants found in the food and drink we consume daily. Brochantite ignites curiosity, intuition and creativity making it the ideal talisman for students of all kinds. The warm energy emanating from Brochantite soothes those suffering from emotional trauma and a restless mind and works to replace feelings of fear guilt and worry with feelings of contentment and peace. This beautiful green stone resonates strongly with the Heart Chakra and massively boosts intuitive abilities and even clairvoyance, especially when using alongside other stones such as Bustamite, Lolite and Rainbow Moonstone.

Legend has it that a Brochantite crystal will lose its lustre and shine as a pre-warning of deceit, upcoming danger or if traitors are nearby.
Colour
Green
Black
Birthstone
August
Zodiac
Capricorn
Energetic Frequencies
Chakras
The Heart Chakra
Carnelian
Carnelian is a stone found in India as well as South America and exists in red/orange hues with deep red being the most desirable. This stone is a known as one of the stones of motivation and for having strong connections to bravery, courage and physical power which can help the shy and introverted in taking on leadership roles and in becoming engaging and eloquent public speakers. The name carnelian comes from the Latin word for

'flesh. In Ancient Egypt, Carnelian was known as 'the setting sun', with its orange form holding female energetic frequencies with the red gemstones being associated with male energies. Carnelian is an energy-boosting stone that acts as a link between our emotional state and inner-self guiding users towards greater levels of independence. As a healing stone Carnelian is thought to aid the body in absorbing minerals and nutrients, improves and maintains blood flow, pressure and circulation, clears congestion, cures haemorrhoids, heals bad backs, joint pain, arthritis, scars, and even improve fertility. This gemstone acts as a stabiliser stone brings the user into the present, which is great for daydreamers and worriers alike as well as making a perfect talisman for those who find themselves lacking in concertation and motivation. It is also said to increase the appetite. Carnelian in both of its main colours carries close links to both Sacral (orange hues) and Base Chakras (red hues) that provides the wearer with enhanced

intuition (gut instinct) emotional stability and an air of joy and friendship.
Colour
Red/Orange
Pink
Brown
Birthstone
May
July
August
Zodiac
Aries
Taurus
Virgo
Planet
Mars
Energetic Frequencies
Creativity
Healing
Power
Chakras
The Second or Sacral Chakra
The Base or Root Chakra
Celestite

A crystal with colourings of clear blue tropical seas, Celestite is a relatively modern stone with it being first reported in the late 1700s. It is known for its celestial blue hues but can also appear extremely pale, white, clear, yellow, and light reds. The appearance of Celestite would suggest its energy is light and subtle, however, the vibrational frequencies displayed by Celestite and their effects are both influential and powerful. Keeping a piece of Celestite in the North corner of your bedroom will establish it as an uplifting and relaxing space and as Celestite's 'water-energy' fills the space it will become a tranquil space perfect for prayer, rest, and contemplation. It is said that Celestite can ignite latent psychic abilities and has been used by Wiccans, psychics, spiritualists, and healers to enhance all manner of abilities from clairvoyance and telepathy to remote reviewing and telekinesis. Celestite activates all three of the higher chakras, the Crown, Third Eye, and Throat Chakras filling us with light energy, providing us with insight and inspiring us with truth and strengthening our fortitude in order to allow us to stay on the correct path. This is one of the few stones that is also directly linked to the Eighth Chakra known as the Soul Star Chakra, the only chakra that is located outside of the body and is permanently linked to the earth's energy field and is thought to play a significant role in the process of enlightenment through its links to spiritual entities and by opening the doors to divine knowledge. It is a stone that compliments and accentuates the qualities of other crystals such as the Quartz family, Moldavite, and Pollucite. Celestite is known to expand the conscious and balances emotions; however, it also cleanses both body and aura and stimulates the body's natural detoxification processes. It has been used in the treatment of ear, eye and throat infections and is also thought to be beneficial to those in recovery from head or brain injury. The energy emitted by Celestite works wonders for stress and persistent general pain, its vibrations penetrate and sooth the body calming the muscles, stabilising heart rate and stomach functions. As a talisman Celestite acts a dispeller crystal which energises the body as it purges and negative emotional build up that may be blocking the chakras or aura. It relieves unnecessary worry, excessive guilt, and irrational fears by redirecting misused energy and attention towards more positive aspects of our lives, making Celestite invaluable as it is enchanting.

Colour
Light Blue
White
Clear
Yellow
Red
Birthstone
February
March
Zodiac
Cancer
Gemini
Energetic Frequencies

Protection
Healing
Magic
Transformation
Tranquillity
Chakras
The Crown Chakra
The Third Eye Chakra
The Throat Chakra
The Soul Star Chakra
Citrine

Citrine's name is derived from the French word citron meaning 'lemon' but is also regularly known as both the Merchant's Stone due to its uncanny ability to increase bank balances, and the Stone of the Mind due to the ancient belief that placing a Citrine stone on the forehead can activate the users latent psychic abilities. Natural Citrine is a pure and radiant yellow, sometimes containing translucent golden hues which emanate energetic frequencies that ground negative energy and create an environment which attracts only the best and most jovial of moods. It is thought that Citrine assists in the removal of bodily toxins and helps in maintaining a healthy digestive system. It is also thought to aid in blood circulation, blood detoxification, and in maintaining a healthy thyroid. Citrine is primarily a happy stone that works to eliminate fear and inadequacy from the user's life and replaces it with courage, fortitude, and clarity of thought. It holds associations with the Crown, Solar Plexus and Sacral Chakra and boasts the ability to realign, balance, and stimulate the chakra network allowing for a better synthesis between body and mind which boosts the immune system as well as our creativity and overall intellectual and psychic talents. Citrine is a great stone for meditation and is one of the 'Seeker Stones' which when used as a talisman can change lives by guiding the user towards new horizons like a compass guiding us in the direction of fresh knowledge and fresh starts.

Colour
Yellow with Dark Brown Hues
Birthstone
November

Zodiac
Cancer
Gemini
Leo
Planet
Jupiter
Energetic Frequencies
Money
Healing
Luck
Defence
Chakras
The Crown Chakra
The Sacral Chakra
The Solar Plexus Chakra

Datolite

Datolite is a crystal that displays a wide range of colour hues, in Datolite's case due to the varying silver, iron oxide, and copper contained within each individual stone. With colourings ranging from warm pink and reds to peach, greens, violet and purple, Datolite is a highly collectable to Reiki experts, spiritual practitioners and even specialist such as mineralogists. Datolite is well known as a stone that inspires acceptance, love and affection. It is said that wearing Datolite will increase the wearer's attractiveness and also act to solidify and strengthen already existing relationships by adding new depths of understanding. Around the home, it works well for calming squabbling siblings, rivalries and soothes built up emotions and frustrations acting to diffuse arguments by filling the room with its peaceful energy. Datolite helps to balance unruly emotions, making it popular among spiritualists and healers. Its vibrations permeate the aura, releasing any pent up anxiety, excessive guilt and fear, and gently replaces it with feelings of contentment and peace. Datolite has strong connections to the mind enhancing logic and problem-solving abilities as well as memory retention, creativity and understanding making it the perfect stone for those studying as it also adds a certain fluidity to thoughts allowing them to flow fast and freely giving way to new insights and bursts of inspiration. The vibrational energy of Datolite is exceptionally high and has a particularly strong resonance with the Third Eye and Crown Chakra which, through practice alongside meditation is known to facilitate astral projection and other out of body experiences like past life regression and remote viewing. It is a very popular stone for those wishing to activate or amplify any innate psychic abilities. Datolite directly links the ethereal and physical bodies, particularly the energy of the heart and mind. This results in powerful transformative and healing energies that affect us both physically and emotionally. These energies help us to accept and move beyond past traumas as well as helping us to deal with current conflicts that may be causing stress and worry. The very same healing energies support the body's natural ability to create insulin and furthermore it works to maintain healthy blood sugar levels. Datolite stimulates proper nerve function and is believed to also shorten recovery time from any never related damage or illnesses. It helps the body to deal with bodily issues relating to quitting smoking, drugs, alcohol or prescribed medication and so is a useful crystal for recovering drug addicts. This crystal is one that activates the entire chakra network, aligning and opening the individual chakras to allow for the free flow of energy throughout the body bringing vitality and freshness to the body as a whole and as such makes Datolite an essential stone for crystal and mineral enthusiasts of all kinds.

Colour
Pink
Red
Peach
Green
Violet
Purple
Birthstone
March
April
Zodiac
Aries
Energetic Frequencies
Healing
Transformative

Love
Chakras
The Crown Chakra
The Third Eye Chakra
The Solar Plexus Chakra

Chapter 10: More Than 380 Different Conditions And Their Healing Crystals

The chart laid out in this chapter guides novice users of crystals with regards to what stone is proper for different ailments:

CONDITIONS	HEALING CRYSTAL
Abdomen	Smoky Quartz
Abdominal colic	Mother of pearl
Absent-mindedness	Carnelian
Abundance	Amber
Accidents	Tiger Eye
Aches	Rose Quartz
Acid Indigestion	Varicite
Acidity	Green jasper
Acne	Amethyst
Addictions	Dumortierite
Aggression	Carnelian
Air Purification	Quartz Crystal

Air travel stress	Hematite
Alcoholism	black onyx
Allergies	Aquamarine
Allergies to pollen	Chrysocolla
Ambition	Morganite
Amplification of energy	Rock Quartz
Analytical qualities	Agate
Ancient Wisdom	Quartz Crystal
Anemia	Garnet
Angel Communication	Selenite
Anger	Carnelian
Angina	Dioptase
Anorexia	Topaz
Anxiety	Azurite-Malachite
Appendix	Chrysolite
Arthritis	Abalone
Artistic Expression	Botswana Agate

Artistic growth	Blue topaz
Asthma	Amber
Astral Projection	Ametrine
Astrology	Angelite
Attention Deficit Disorder	Sodalite
Attraction	Sunstone
Attuning to the Earth	Chrysocolla
Aura balancing	Rutilated Quartz
Aura Cleansing	Crystal Quartz
Autism	Sugilite
Awareness	Picture Jasper
Back issues	Petrified wood
Backache	Blue Agate
Bad temper	Green Aventurine
Balance	Tourmalinated Quartz
Balancing Relationships	Peridot
Baldness	Aquamarine

Banish Grief	Black Onyx
Beauty	Amber
Biliousness	Jasper
Bitterness	Agate
Bladder	Red Jasper
Bladder trouble	Bloodstone
Bleeding	Clear Quartz
Blessing	Jade
Blood	Carnelian
Blood circulation	Fire Agate
Blood cleansing	Amethyst
Blood clotting	Hematite
Blood diseases	Amethyst
Blood poisoning	Carnelian
Blood pressure	Aventurine
Boils	Sapphire
Bone marrow	Chalcedony
Bones	Obsidian
Bowels	Jasper
Brain	Lapis Lazuli
Brain tonic	Carnelian
Bravery	Agates
Breathlessness	Black Onyx

Bronchitis	Red Jasper
Bruises	Carnelian
Burns	Sodalite
Calcium deficiencies	Amazonite
Calming	Silver Grey Moonstone
Calming of body	Blue Topaz
Calmness of mind	Agate
Cancer	Carnelian
Cancer related diseases	Rhodochrosite
Catarrh	Blue Agate
Cell rejuvenation	Sodalite
Central nervous system	Rock Crystal
Cervix	Zoisite
Chakras balanced	Quartz Crystal
Chakras opened	Fluorite
Change	Snowflake

balancing	Obsidian
Changing habits	Tiger Eye
Cheerfulness	Tourmaline
Chest pains	Malachite
Childbirth	Peridot
Circulation	Carnelian
Circulatory problems	Rhodochrosite
Clairaudience	Malachite
Clairvoyance	Chrysoprase
Cleansing	Sunstone
Coldness deflection	Topaz
Colds	Fluorite
Colic	Malachite
Color blindness	Amethyst
Comfort	Gold Calcite
Communication	Turquoise
Compassion	Chrysoprase
Concentration	Carnelian
Connection in general	Turquoise

Connection with God	Marcasite
Constipation	Citrine
Contentment	Amethyst
Convulsions	Quartz Crystal
Cough	Aquamarine
Courage	Sunstone Tiger Iron
Cramp	Amethyst
Creativity	Blue Topaz
Crown energy	Rock Crystal
Decision Making	Aventurine
Depression	Chrysoprase
Depression	Tiger Eye
Despair	Carnelian
Diabetes	Rock Crystal
Diarrhea	Malachite
Digestion	Peridot
Direction	Citrine
Dizziness	Lapis Lazuli
Doubt	staurolite
Dream inducer	Garnet
Dreams	Sugilite

Dreams manifestation	Amber
Dream intuitiveness	Jade
Drunkenness	Amethyst
Ear internal issues	Rhodonite
Ear problems	Blue Agate
Ear trouble	Sapphire
Earache	Amber
Eczema	Green Aventurine
Edema	Amethyst
Ego detachment	Citrine
Elixir of life	Sodalite
Emotional balance	Aventurine
Emotional distance	Blue Topaz
Emotional energy	Garnet
Emotional strength	Rose Quartz
Emotions	Moonstone

calming	
Emotions negativity	Peridot
Emotional blockage	Blue Tourmaline
Endocrine system	magnetite
Endurance	Sodalite
Energy	Red Tiger Eye
Energy of body	Petrified Wood
Energy booster	Amethyst
Epilepsy	Jasper
Eye disorders	Magnetite
Eyes	Aquamarine
Eye watering	Onyx
Eyesight	Obsidian Snowflake
Eyesight weakness	Topaz
Eyestrain	Emerald
Fainting	Lapis Lazuli
Faith	Pearls
Fallopian	Chrysoprase

tubes	
Falls	Tourmaline
Fatigue	Ruby
Fear	Diamond
Fear	Snowflake Obsidian
Fertility	Rock Crystal
Fever	Aventurine
Fever reduction	Ruby
Fire Energy	Amber
Focus	Black Onyx
Forgetfulness	Emerald
Forgiveness	Rhodochrosite
Fractures	Mother of pearl
Friendship	Peridot
Frustration	Howlite
Gall bladder	Orange Calcite
Gardening	Moss Agate
General health tonic	Green Aventurine
Generosity	Rhodonite

Glands	Blue Lace Agate
Goiter	Amber
Good luck	Moonstone
Grief	Obsidian clear
Grounding	Unakite
Grounding Earth Energy	Aventurine
Hair	Rock Crystal
Hair problems	Obsidian
Happiness	Malachite
Hay fever	Tiger Eye
Headache	Moonstone
Healing emotional wounds	Green Amber
Healing generally	Quartz Crystal
Hearing	Rhodonite
Heart disease	Carnelian
Heart trouble	Dioptase
Heartburn	Peridot
Hemorrhage	Chrysoprase
Hemorrhoids	Sulphur
Hips	Petrified

	Wood
Hostility	Grossular
Humility	Sunstone
Humility	Chrysoprase
Hypertension	Apatite
Hypochondria	Tiger Eye
Idealism	Bloodstone
Imagination	Sapphire
Immune deficiency	Sugilite
Immune system	Snow Quartz
Impotence	Rhodonite
Independence	Blue Aventurine
Indigestion	Citrine
Infection	Amber
Infection defense	Garnet
Infertility	Coral
Inflammation	Carnelian
Influenza	Pyrite
Inner Child	Carnelian
Insomnia	Zircon
Inspiration	Tourmaline

Intellect	Emerald
Intellectual stimulation	Blue Aventurine
Intestinal disorders	Amber
Intuitive awareness	Turquoise
Irritated throat	Rhodonite
Itching	Green Aventurine
Jealousy	Peridot
joints	Ruby
Judgment	Labradorite
Kidney stones	Malachite
Kidneys	Bloodstone
Kindness	Chrysoprase
Knees	Mother of pearl
Knowledge	Rock Crystal
Laryngitis	Rhodonite
Larynx	Morganite
Learning	Citrine, Jet
Leg cramp	Magnetite
Liver disorders	Rhodonite
Logic	Sodalite

Loneliness	Amethyst
Long life	Moonstone
Longevity	Sodalite
Love	Rose Quartz
Loyalty	Moonstone
Luck	Tiger Eye
Lunar Energy	Labradorite
Lungs	Pyrite
Lymph glands	Tourmaline
Magical Power	Jet
Malaria	Amber
M.E (Fatigue syndrome)	Clear Quartz
Meditation	Turquoise
Melancholy	Carnelian
Memory	Hematite
Menopause	Rose Quartz
Menstrual cycle	Carnelian
Menstrual disorders	Coral
Menstruation	Ruby
Mental breakdown	Smithsonite
Mental Clarity	Turquoise

Mental Cleanser	Malachite
Mental Disorders	Beryl
Mental Power	Selenite
Metabolism, growth	Amazonite
Migraine	Aventurine
Mind	Jasper
Miscarriage	Chrysoprase
Misfortune	Tourmaline
Motor responses	Apatite
Mouth troubles	Sodalite
Multiple sclerosis	Red Jasper
Muscle spasms	Dioptase
Muscles	Hematite
Mysteries of the Universe	Labradorite
Nails	Obsidian
Neck tension	Rose Quartz
Neck strain	Chrysoprase
Negative	Black

energy	Tourmaline
Negative energy	Obsidian Snowflake
Negative vibrations	Green Tourmaline
Negativity release	Tourmalinated Quartz
Nervous system	Alexandrite
Nervousness	Sapphire
Neuralgia	Hematite
New Beginnings	Azurite-Malachite
Night driving	Cat's Eye
Nightmares	Rhodonite
Obesity	Rock Crystal
Obsessions	Black Onyx
Occult powers	Peridot
Opening of heart	Rose Quartz
Optimism	Chalcedony
Osteoporosis	Amazonite
Ovaries	Chrysoprase
Overwhelmed	Agates
Pain	Carnelian

Pain soothing	Ruby
Pain escape	Hematite
Pancreas	Smoky Quartz
Paralysis	Rock Crystal
Passion	Red Tiger Eye
Past-life recall	Selenite
Patience	Chrysoprase
Peace of mind	Sapphire
Peace and harmony	Turquoise
Personal power	Carnelian
Personal willpower	Tiger Iron
Phobias	Obsidian clear
Piles	Heliotrope
Pineal gland	Lazulite
Pituitary	Sugilite
PMS	Moonstone
Pneumonia	Fluorite
Poisoning	Malachite
Poisonous bites	Amazonite
Positive Outlook	Tiger Eye
Power Stones	Earth Stones

Practicality	Turquoise
Pregnancy	Carnelian
Prophecy	Emerald
Prosperity	Turquoise
Prostate	Chrysoprase
Protection	Tiger Eye
Psychic development	Azurite
Psychic Power	Sugilite
Psychic Power	Moldavite
Psychic Protection	Black Obsidian
Psycho-somatic Pain	Bloodstone
Public speaking	Amber
Pulse speed	Hematite
Pulse steadiness	Jasper
Purifier	Smoky Quartz
Quarreling of couples	Rhodonite
Red blood cell	Amethyst
Rejuvenator	Sodalite
Reproductive	Rose Quartz

system	
Resentments	Agates
Respiratory tract	Rhodochrosite
Rheumatism	Copper
Rigid mind	Sodalite
Sadness	Red Jasper
Scalds	Sodalite
Scar tissue	Rock Crystal
Schizophrenia	lepidolite
Sciatica	Hematite
Scientific Outlook	Blue Goldstone
Self discipline	Sunstone
self-knowledge	Citrine
Self-control	Sardonyx
Self-Expression	Blue Aventurine
Self-Image	Galena
Self-love	Rose Quartz
Sensuality	Garnet
Serenity	Aquamarine
Sex improvement	Smoky Quartz
Sexual	Carnelian

appetite	
Shoulder strain	Chrysoprase
Shyness	lepidolite
Sinus	Sulphur
Skin	Corundum
Skin diseases	Garnet
Skin problems	Green Aventurine
Sleep	Howlite
Sleeplessness	Topaz
Smell	Tiger Eye
Solar Energy Stones	Amber
Sores	Green Aventurine
Sorrow eased	Chrysoprase
Spasms	Carnelian
Speech	Rhodonite
Spine strengthening	Obsidian
Spirituality	Amethyst
Spleen strengthening	albite
Stamina	Carnelian

Stammering	Blue Topaz
Stomach	Rhodochrosite
Stomach ulcers	Pyrite
Strength	Tiger Iron
Stress	Grey Moonstone
Stroke	Lapis Lazuli
Success	Tiger Eye
Talent	Bloodstone
Taste	Topaz
Teeth	Calcite
Teeth grinding	Amber
Tension	Carnelian
Testicles	Zoisite
Thinking enhancement	Amazonite
Thought clearing	Celestite

Chapter 11: How To Use Crystals For Healing

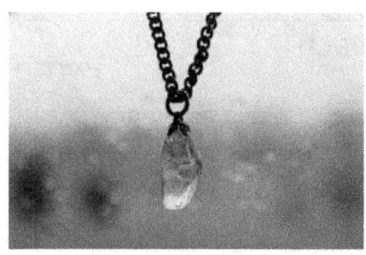

There are many ways you can harness the healing powers of crystals to use it for your needs. This chapter deals with a few such methods and some tips as well.

Program the Crystal with Your Intention

Programming your crystal is empowering it with the energy needed to focus its healing powers on a specific task you have in mind. Programming your crystals with the chosen intent helps to magnify its powers. Also, part of the programming involves dedicating the crystal to some divine power (god, goddess, deity, or the universal power) so that the intensity of the gemstone's functioning is improved.

Use the following steps to program your crystal:
- Make sure the crystal is cleansed and cleared using a suitable method from the list discussed in Chapter Four.
- Then, hold the crystal in your hand and sense its power and energy. After the cleansing process, you will find that the energy of the crystal is more profound and intense than before. You can easily sense its power.
- As you sense and connect with this mysterious and inherent power of the crystal, send up a prayer to your god or any other divine being you have faith in to connect you with the crystal. Remember gemstones behave like living beings and can hear and respond to your requests even if the communication channel is not the one you are used to.
- Once you feel the connection with the core of the crystal, close your eyes and think of the intent that you want to empower it with. Visualize the result in your mind and imagine a streak of white light streaming from this picture moving

towards the crystal. Now, visualize this picture filling every nook and corner of the crystal so that your intent is completely wrapped inside your crystal.

- Now, open your eyes slowly and thank the crystal for agreeing to help you with your needs. Your crystal is programmed with the power of your intention. You can draw its energy whenever you want to move toward your desire.

Another crucial step to programming your crystal is to dedicate it so that no one else can reprogram it intentionally or unintentionally. Here are the steps to dedicate your programmed gemstone to your guardian angel for protection:

- Hold the programmed crystal in your hand and say aloud, 'May only the highest-energy power in this universe use this crystal and its energies.'
- Focus on your crystal intently until you believe your guardian angel has heard you and accepted your request.
- The crystal is now dedicated and protected from misuse.

Meditating with Crystals

One of the biggest paradoxes about meditation is that it is extremely easy to understand and needs no other tool but your body and mind, and yet, mastering the technique can take an entire lifetime. However, there are some tools that can help you hasten the process of learning meditation and also helps you achieve deeper levels of meditation than before. The healing of crystals is one such tool that enhances the power of your meditation. Use the following processes to meditate with crystals:

Choose your gemstone. Many factors have to be included to make the right choice. Some of the elements needed to be factored into your choice if crystals include:

• The frequency of your own vibrational energy; choose a crystal that is aligned with this frequency.

• Your intention; make sure you select that is aligned with your intentions. Do reread Chapters Five and Six to understand which crystal is best for which intention, and then make your choice.

- Sometimes, you might have to use a crystal that magnifies the power of the specific gemstone you have chosen based on the properties. For example, suppose you have chosen rose quartz to attract love and romance in your life, then hold this crystal in one hand, and selenite or clear quartz in the other hand so that the properties of rose quartz are amplified.

Find a suitable place for your meditation session. Make sure it is quiet and undisturbed. If you choose to use a room in your house, then make sure all your electronic devices are either switched off or on silent so that the notifications don't bother you.

Hold the crystals in your hand and restate your intentions. Allow the energy of the crystals to permeate through your body as you hold the gemstones gently. Imagine your intentions resulting in positive outcomes in your mind and allow the healing light from the crystal to light up the picture of your intention. Simply place your faith in your crystals and seek their help unabashedly. You are drawn to crystals because they want to help you.

Now, close your eyes and focus on your breath. Just observe the inflow and outflow of your breath. Every time your mind goes to other thoughts, gently bring back its focus on your breathing.

Mentally scan through your body and release tensions from those parts where you feel stressed out.

Imagine the power of your crystals flowing from the palms of your hand and moving through your body rejuvenating and refreshing every cell.

There is no time limit to this session. You can meditate as long as you wish. When you feel satisfied with your session, then open your eyes slowly, and thank the universal power or your guardian angel and the crystal for participating in the meditation session with you.

Creating Healing Grid or Layouts

Crystal grids are extremely powerful tools to help manifest your intentions, goals, and desires. The primary difference between using a single crystal and a crystal grid is that the latter has the power of a latticed energy network that combines the energy fields of multiple crystals for optimum results. In addition to the combined energies of numerous crystals, the grid also access the sacred power of geometric figures, and your intention, of course.

This combined power of sacred geometry and multiple crystals magnify your intentions no end giving you far more improved results than a single crystal can. The downside is that you cannot create crystal grids for immediate use for which the single crystal is your best option. So, depending on the situation and your need, you can choose between using a crystal or a crystal grid to harness the power and energy of gemstones. You can use the following steps to create a crystal layout or grid:

Things needed to make a grid:

- A suitable, undisturbed location in your home
- A small note with your intention clearly written down on it

- A central crystal that is very effective in directing your intention more powerfully than if you had a grid without a central gemstone
- Tumbled stones with energy fields that synchronize with your intention
- A quartz crystal to activate the grid

A cloth to lay out the crystal grid; even though this element is optional and you can create a grid on the floor or a table, most healers opine that using a cloth enhances the power of the grid.

- The first step of making crystal grid is to know and understand your intention. What is the purpose of your grid? Do you want to get rid of negative energies? Do you want to bring in good fortune and abundance into your life? Do you need a boost in creativity?
- Find out your intention and make a note of this in that small piece of paper. Choosing your intention is very important because it will affect the selection of your crystals. For example, if you are looking for wealth and abundance, then you must select 'wealth' crystals like aventurine,

pyrite, citrine, etc. And yet, remember there are no right or wrong crystals to choose from. Trust your instincts and pick up those gemstones that you are drawn to.

• Cleanse the space on which you want to create your grid by smudging with sage or any other cleansing process discussed in Chapter Four.

• Fold the paper on which you have written your specific intention. Place it in the center of the grid cloth.

• Now, close your eyes, breathe deeply, and state your intention loudly. Alternately, you can visualize your intention in your mind.

• Next, start placing the crystals around the paper with your intention written on it. Start from the outermost layer, and move inwards until you reach the paper. Remember to focus on your intention as you place each stone in the grid.

• Lastly, place the central crystal on the paper that has your written intention.

• The next step is to activate the grid using the quartz crystal point. For this, take the quartz crystal and draw imaginary lines connecting all the crystals on the grid. This process connects the stones energetically to each other. You can pretend you are playing that kid game called 'connect the dots'.

With this process, your grid activated and its healing energy has started its work. To enhance the power of your crystal grid, you can place candles and other energy-enhancing tools around the grid.

Making Crystal Essences and Elixirs

Creating and using gem essences are wonderful methods used to gain the healing powers of a specific crystal. The gemstone is put into purified water. This highly vibrated water is allowed to capture the gemstone meanings and the crystal's healing properties. They offer the body rejuvenating energy. This water works similar to mineral springs, which was used for centuries to heal, both, internally and externally. Gem essences are meant to stabilize all of the energy centers within your body.

Gem essences are very simple to make at home. While choosing your crystals to make the gem essences, it is recommended that you choose those, which have similar gemstone meanings and properties so that your intention for the healing stones would be the same. For instance, if you want to include love energy in your life, the first thing a person would think of would be a beautiful flower like a rose which resembles love. Keeping this in mind, you can create a Rose Quartz essence. Also, you must remember to thoroughly cleanse the crystal before using it or preparing any sort of crystal essence to relieve it of any pollutants or negative energy.

The process to prepare crystal essence is fairly simple. All you need is a clear glass jar, preferably with a lid and your crystals, which have been fully exposed to either the sun or the full moon. Doing so cleanses the crystals and makes them ready for use.

To begin, hold your crystals in both hands and state your intention. Your intention can either be visualized or can be said out loud. Additionally, you can state the benefits, which you hope to receive after the crystal healing process out loud. Doing so helps transfer the intentions from the crystal to the essence directly. You may seek guidance of God and do multiple breathing exercises to clear the mind of all negativity to boost the healing process.

Place the crystals at the bottom of the glass container and fill it with purified water (preferably alkaline). Close the lid to the glass jar and place the entire setup out in the sun for 2-4 hours, allowing it to charge. The jar can also be placed for 24 hours so that the essence can get its full share of sunlight as well as moonlight. However, this method could be dangerous if the chosen crystals have components which, when used in excess become toxic. It is recommended that you store the remaining elixir in the refrigerator.

Once this is done, be cautious around the crystals. If you spend too much time around them or have any sort of direct, physical contact with them, your energy tampers with that of the crystal, which minimizes the overall healing effect.

There are multiple ways in which a person can use the essence he or she has prepared. Some people like to put a few drops of it directly on their skin, neck or even in their tongue everyday. Others like to put it in the beverages, which they drink during the day so that they can have the essence at occasional shifts.

For the best benefits, it is recommended that the essence is mixed with shampoo or body lotion, which the person uses while bathing. In this manner, they get cleaned externally as well as internally. For a positive start to their day, people put their essence in spritzer bottles and spray it on their face after waking up.

Rose Quartz essence is known to open up a person's heart to love, happiness and forgiveness. It makes the consumer compassionate and friendly and also balances emotions to bring about inner peace and harmony.

Benefits of Using Crystal Essence - Different benefits are obtained on consuming different crystal essences. For example, quartz crystals are able to store, focus and amplify energy and enhance spiritual growth and wisdom. The Moonstone is a very personal stone and brings about success in love and business matters. It is believed to be the most powerful and effective during a full moon night. Moonstone helps receive advice from the subconscious mind to calm a person down and balance their emotions.

Pink Tourmaline is believed to bring about peace and acceptance and love to oneself. Its effect is termed 'Aphrodisiac', named after the Greek God of love, Aphrodite. It is believed to transform negative energy into positive energy. Desert Rose Selenite helps in clearing the mind of any negative energy.

Ametrine is very useful to sustain long and prolonged illnesses as it brings the consumer aware of the cause for his or her disease. It also helps in reducing stress and stimulates creativity. Blue Aragonite is good for teaching people patience and for those who are too hard on themselves. It balances emotions and cleanses any blockages in the heart or throat.

Amethyst is widely used for spiritual growth and reduce addictions to drugs and alcohol. Lepidolite is specifically used to reduce depression and stress and is supposed to bring a good future for the consumer.

Tibetan Quartz Crystal is one of the 12 Master crystals as it is very powerful. It helps in recalling dreams and helps a person meditate. It is also known as the 'feel good' stone as it improves physical energy, strength and stamina.

Blue Lace Agate is a stone with soft energy. It brings about a cool and calm effect. Its primary function is to bring about peace of mind. Along with its cooling effect, it reduces deep anger, resentment, and anxiety. If you have to fight a hard battle, in your personal or professional life, it is recommended that you consume the essence of Blue Lace Agate to go well prepared for whatever lies ahead. It also helps a person to understand himself or herself.

Prehnite is another crystal essence, which is used for enhancing spiritual growth. It helps a person visualizing what he or she wants. It is useful for prolonged meditation. To get rid of any negative or hurtful past experiences, people consume essences of this stone to 'declutter' their minds for them to move on,

Create a Sacred Space in Your Home

You can harness the power of energy crystals by creating a sacred space or altar in your home. In fact, sacred spaces at home are becoming increasingly popular as many people use this consecrated place to do their yoga or meditation without any disturbance.

Designing a sacred space in your home using crystals will act as a reminder to move towards your intention each time you take a peek or walk along this space. You can make a crystal grid in your sacred space, and rearrange the grid each time you want a new intention realized with the power of crystals.

Other Ways of Using Crystals

You can simply carry your favorite crystals in your pocket or purse. Remember that some gemstones are extra brittle and soft, and if you handle them in a wild way, you could damage them.

You can add crystals to your bath and allow the healing powers to seep into your body through the pores on your skin. Of course, not all crystals should be put in water, and therefore, do your research well before adding any gemstone to your bath water.

You can simply place energy-giving crystals in any living space including your bedroom, living room, study, kitchen, or your office. Here are some ideas of which crystal works best for which room:

Crystals for your bedroom - Three crystals that are great for your bedroom are amethyst, black tourmaline, and obviously rose quartz. The auric energies of each of these crystals helps to build love, intimacy, and an improved relationship with your beloved.

Crystals for the living room - Selenite is a great crystal for the living room, and so is apophyllite. Although this book does not discuss in detail, it is enough to know that both selenite and apophyllite promote openness, transparency, and honesty so that family members can bond with each other without fear or uncertainty.

Crystals for the kitchen - If there is one crystal that is perfect for your kitchen, then it must be carnelian for its ability to build creativity by opening up your sacral chakra. And no other place in the house needs creativity as much as your kitchen considering that you have to whip up delicious and nutritious meals for your family on a daily basis.

Crystals for the dining area - Turquoise is a great crystal to place in the dining area as it helps in creating healthy and conscious eating habits. Citrine placed in the dining area helps to infuse your dining space and the eating experience with happiness and joy.

Crystals for office space - Use pyrite in your working space or office space to get focus and clarity of thought to ensure you make informed choices that positively affects your decision-making and professional skills.

And finally, you can make beautiful jewelry with your favorite crystals and wear them on your body. Not only do you access to its healing powers but also get to enhance your physical profile by adding oomph and oeuvre to your personality.

The healing power of crystals can be harnessed in multiple different ways. You can choose the method depending on the availability of space, ease of use, and other factors that are unique to your lifestyle and needs.

CHAPTER 12: COMPLETE CRYSTAL FROM A TO Z

Letting crystals into your lives enables you to adopt old and mystical wisdom—but you also need the means to comprehend these rocks as they are today.

With our advice on your part, you will discover out all you need to learn about the healing crystals for spiritual growth.

Crystal Meanings

Abalone Shell

Alongside its marvelous ocean of colors, it is a protective rock, not least because it performs the same literal purpose in nature. At moments when your trust seems to be giving up, or you think uncomfortable, achieve your Abalone Shell for convenience and instruction.

This makes this stone popular in overcoming anxieties, but also in remaining true to oneself –particularly in issues of the core. If you sometimes discover that anxiety and self-sabotage are going to get in the manner of your interactions, this might be a rock for you.

Agate

Agate has been heralded for millennia as a rock of notable equilibrium and grounding energy. There is a good feeling of positivity within Agate, which implies that even the most skeptical of us can discover some hope for the future to let in the forces of this stone.

Agate functions because it links you to a wider view and allows you to see the pros and cons of any specified scenario, which makes it a nice rock for those of us wishing to join a fresh chapter in life—a fresh connection, a fresh career change and so on—securely and confidently.

Amazonite

There is an extensive amount of love and healing energy in the Amazon that can assist break the cycles of adverse ideas that you may be facing in your lives. In particularly pronounced instances, Amazonite can even assist in revealing and breaking through the karmic models of past incarnations and lifetimes.

Amazonite is often seen as a rock of courage–appropriate, perhaps, to be deemed Amazonian warriors! It can awaken you to your bravery and assist you in taking a position assertively, but compassionately, by breaking the illusions that keep you on a loop of errors, repeated all over again.

Amethyst

Always a guiding light for psychic professionals and a lovely crystal for use in jewelry, Amethyst is both common and strong.

It can awaken you to greater wisdom and link you advise from beyond the physical globe, but it is just as efficient as a rock for physical therapy. In addition to its capacity to ameliorate headaches and joint pain, Amethyst also carries a feeling of peace.

Because of this, it's a nice crystal to decrease mental pressure and to stop your brain from concentrating on the same thoughts of uneasiness repeatedly, disturbing sleep and concentration.

Apatite

Ambition and a feeling of life-enthusiasm are all enhanced when the emotions of Apatite are allowed into yourself. This stone is colored in a wonderful shade that enhances the clarity of your mind. It can be fascinating to look at.

Apatite is regarded as a nice rock for creative thinking, meaning that it is not only useful for those who operate in the press and the arts but also that it unlocks fresh, innovative ideas for researchers and business-minded individuals. This is a flexible rock, with plenty to give to all fields of existence.

Apophyllite

With its frosty white and cool blue hues, Apophyllite is a wonderful rock to calm an overactive mind. It can also assist avoid over-energized poor habits, such as nervous twitches and tics.

Apophyllite, though, is a rock that is as much about avoidance as it is about a remedy. It operates by putting to light the root causes of certain activities and bad habits of lives. It may not be necessarily a pleasant method, but it is essential for spiritual growth and fresh stages of soul development. This stone, too, helps to alleviate the strain of these changes.

Aquamarine

As the name suggests, Aquamarine is a rock that is extremely bound to water and its beauty, nutritious characteristics. You may well think that the core of existence itself awaits you in this rock, so powerful that it's cleansing powers can often be.

But this is also a rock about the tides of transition in life. When you have difficulty getting away from challenging circumstances and interactions, Aquamarine connects you to your internal power. It can also assist you in positioning yourself with other individuals on the same trip.

Aventurine

Aventurine is a stone that is tightly linked to the Heart Chakra and that's where some ancient sayings about pursuing one's soul are born. Harmonizing with the adventurous vibrating nature of this crystal, these ideas encourage you to follow your heart with boldness!

There is a sense of playful risk involved with Aventurine. Many have named it the Gambler's Stone, thinking that it links you with nice luck and fortunate spots. While luck is perceived differently by every individual, it hardly hurts a little opportunity to come one way!

Azurite

Azurite is often referred to as the Stone of the Heavens, making it a common option for those who seek to adopt divine advice and ties to the angelic domain. This precious stone helps to open one's mind to what a solely pragmatic mind would find impossible.

It's a rock of faith and belief in a divine figure. However, it also encourages self-confidence with just as much power and it can assist you to keep up with vibrant thoughts as and when they hit, proud of your achievement. This crystal also helps to remove stress and concern.

Black Tourmaline

Same as many stones that share its density and color, Black Tourmaline is a guardian stone that protects you from adverse energy.

The crystal has, therefore, become particularly famous with individuals who are naturally empathic, or otherwise capable of absorbing the feelings and energy of others. Black Tourmaline is a powerful barricade to protect you from turmoil or emotional blackmail. It's a true supporter of trust!

However, the more you learn to operate with its energy, the more the crystal becomes useful to safeguard areas and other individuals.

Bloodstone

Despite its possibly provocative title, Bloodstone is very much in your hand, as you'll find out if you begin operating on crystal healing with it. It might help to relieve all sorts of body pain and injuries, or to elevate the effective circulation of blood and through the energy centers of your spiritual body.

Bloodstone is in direct connection to the root Chakra, which is the one that holds you most in physical truth. This is a rock to enjoy the moment, then and experience the pleasures of life. Nevertheless, when utilized in meditation, it becomes a precious anchoring stone that keeps you from going too far into the ethereal domain.

Blue Lace Agate

This is a calming and serene crystal, even if one looks at its colors alone. This stone has a mystical appearance and a lot of depth in the manner light performs even the easiest part of it.

It is linked to your capacity to shape and articulate your thoughts. If you often discover yourself overthinking and criticizing yourself for not taking up against unfair situations declining favors that you ask you to understand are too far-reaching, this crystal can assist you.

It's going to inspire firm but compassionate words that get your point across and it's going to help you see that most people making such requests don't try to be unkind to you.

Bronzite

While the majority of these stones specialize in one specific Chakras, Bronzite is one of the more unique crystals, able to bond with all of your Chakras. It puts them into balance and helps you figure out which parts of yourself most need healing and attention.

Bronzite, however, is a rock that also has many protective characteristics. It enables you to acknowledge when individuals are attempting to take the wool over your eyes and it is also great in triggering the greater components of your immune system. The feared office bug unexpectedly appearing out of nowhere could impact you less frequently!

Carnelian

The vibrant orange of Carnelian might sound like the warmth of sunset, but this is one rock that leaves you all but weary. There is a powerful undercurrent of vitality in this rock that perks you and electrifies your mind with thoughts and aspirations.

Carnelian is also linked to your sacred Chakra, where many pleasures of life are experienced and handled. If your "joie de vivre" is lower than the usual, Carnelian is the stone you need to reinvigorate your lust for life and you're chomping to the point of success.

Celestite

Exploring beyond our physical bodies becomes even easier when Celestite is around us. This rock seems to many to be a direct line to the sky themselves and in the same way, under the forces of this stone, you can relate much more simply to your higher self.

Celestite is the precious stone that is forevermore attracted to those who actively lead a spiritualistic existence, seeking reality, helping the poor, exercising altruism and meditating regularly. However, it also enables those who are just going out on their soul to discover their spiritual legs without feeling daunted.

Chrysocolla

As far as conversion is concerned, it is generally either our goal or the occurrences of existence that force us to alter—sometimes with or without our permission! But regarding Chrysocolla, with divine guidance, you will find that you are able to stimulate constructive change in your life.

This gemstone, with its wealthy earth colors also establishes a wonderful connection with nature. Same as seasons follow their cycle, you will be able to understand the rhythm of your life—and feel empowered to either cherish or interrupt the cycles according to your needs.

Chrysoprase

Although a plain pale green rock may appear, at first sight, Chrysoprase has many concealed depths. In reality, it could be said that this is a perfect stone for digging deeper into your soul too.

This is a rock of reality and enlightenment, which means that besides seeing the lies of others, you will also prevent involving yourself in certain fields of existence. By virtue of the powerful matters of compassion and love that dissipate the energies of this crystal, it is wonderful for mending and conquering traumas.

Citrine

Vibrant in color and also in its energies, Citrine is a gemstone that cannot assist but stimulate positivity and determination. It binds to your solar plexus Chakra, which is where most of the power transfer between individuals truly takes place, as well as some intuitive perspectives—or' good emotions,' as we often call them.

But in addition to enhancing these components of ourselves, Citrine also encourages the concept of development, including personal growth, the progress of a partnership, the evolution of an economic surplus—whatever you concentrate your forces towards.

Citrine boosts your trust appropriately, too, so if you've been feeling on your back foot recently, switch to this crystal to assist you in getting back on track and getting prepared to talk to your item.

Clear Quartz

Look no further than the very title of this crystal to comprehend its hidden healing strength. In other words, Clear Quartz operates by adding simplicity to all around you, allowing you to see the reality of stuff. Luckily, when these truths are a bit hideous or difficult to manage, this crystal also has relaxing energies that stop you from getting too harmed.

Clear Quartz is capable of healing the body and mind with equivalent smoothness, but its specialty is perception—both physical and mental. If you've been suffering from brain fog, or if you've had a confused mind owing to the stress you've experienced, this stone can make things straight for you, providing you a wider view on what to do.

Dalmatian Jasper

Sweet and speckled, Dalmatian Jasper is a precious stone of pure playful energy. If you've somehow forgotten the little joys of life, or you don't seem to have fun in anything you do, this crystal can reinforce your more frantic side.

This glass also enables you to meet the difficulties that come into your lives with a sense of humor—even the wisest of spiritualists understand how strong such a thing can be in the play of life! Dalmatian Jasper gives you a spring in your step and a joy in your heart, but don't worry—it won't leave you spaced out, either.

Dumortierite

Nowadays, everything seems to have to be instant and it can cause even the best of us to have some irrational aspirations. Good things come to those who wait and Dumortierite understands it. Use this crystal to help you see the larger voyage we're all going on and not to sweat the little things.

But in addition to patience, this crystal also encourages fulfillment and the capacity to react deftly to unpredictable modifications in lives. This rock will also reveal the interactions around you that are pulling you down and any toxic factors in your lives will discover their real colors revealed for all to see.

Fluorite

The vivid colors of Fluorite create it a famous stone in its own right, but it is the soothing characteristics of this rock that have made it so well-known. In an age characterized by stress and anxiety disorders, this crystal is a welcome, relaxing relief for the spirit.

Fluorite is a common meditation aid, not least because the state of extreme calm and quietness of mind is so essential for joining the meditative state. However, it may also be helpful if you have trouble sleeping. Just place it under your pillow.

Fuchsite

The majority of healers see Fuchsite as a rock of hard love. While it is invaluable to pierce through illusions, dispel bad karmic models and otherwise break up anything that holds you away, it does this with an energy that is very direct and touching.

However, the data and knowledge that this stone can assist you in relating to are far more important than any mollycoddling–and by being aware of the power of this stone, you will be able to recognize lies and deceit long before they have the opportunity to do any damage.

Garnet

Garnet is popular for being a wealthy purple color and in the same way, this crystal can arouse a warm red enthusiasm. But it's not just about love and it's about enthusiasm for anything else in life that you enjoy—art, practice, leisure, or hobbies.

Garnet helps to encourage you to take advantage of every day and it can assist to cure you physically so that you have the strength and energy to do just that. If you've felt a little caught in a rut, a gemstone can motivate you to stir stuff up in a favorable manner.

Goldstone

It makes sense, of course, that individuals who seek their luck often depend on the energies of Goldstone. It attracts abundance as well as curiosity and it also has a sense of excellent luck. With Goldstone in your hands, you can't assist but feel like there's a large windfall around the corner!

It is a stone of optimism that we could all be confronted with in today's globe of adverse media bias and ever-increasing difficulties before us as a community. Goldstone helps you to find the inner spark of brilliance within you and also gives you the ability to become a force, attracting positive changes around you.

Green Calcite

If you are interested in getting back into harmony with nature, or if you're attempting to discover methods to escape the folly of big city life, Green Calcite can only demonstrate a ticket. It's got this magical value of creating life easy just a little—just enough to take some precious time for you to sit on the beach or stroll through the park.

Green Calcite reminds us all that rest are as essential as curiosity and achievement when it relates to life's progress. Meditation with this crystal also awakens you to the patterns that direct a lot of lives and through this method you can comprehend your cyclical nature.

Hematite

The shiny shine of Hematite may well help to enhance your steely strength, but it also reinforces your physical body. This implies that it allows you to conquer sickness and injury, but it also provides you higher resilience to disease and fatigue.

Hematite focuses the mind and the heart of what is real, tangible, physical and attainable. If you find your head too often in the clouds, or even if your dreams at night are so intense that you are shocked to wake up, this rock can offer you precious grounding energy.

Jade

Crystals that are wealthy in culture and folklore are not much better recognized than Jade. Its link to the Aztecs and ancient China is well known and mythology has been around this rock for thousands of years.

Jade's reputation for safety, inspiration, motivation and healing is just as precise today. This is a lovely, flexible and extremely sought-after rock and its energy and beauty only seem to grow with era.

Jade provides wisdom and abundance to those ready to operate with his talents and he can open your eyes to the inherent duality of existence.

K2 Stone

Named for the pinnacle of the Himalayas, K2 Stone is equally eager to assist you rise to fresh heights. It is, in reality, a mixture of rocks mingled together and its colors are like a vivid summer sky.

This rock is said to amplify one's capacity to withstand the hard circumstances of existence. Sometimes, no matter how many crystals we may use, we will find ourselves unable to change the bad situation the moment we need it. Instead, we need to go through the process to its completion before we can finish it.

Similarly, in terms of physical therapy and wellness, this crystal demonstrates to us that some medical circumstances need to be taught to live with.

Kambaba Jasper

There is an almost animalistic value to Kambaba Jasper, particularly in its appearance. This precious stone talks to the more primordial components of ourselves and promotes us to understand that some items are just a component of human nature.

Of course, there is still every reason to try enlightenment and to go beyond ourselves in spite of that. But Kambaba Jasper will assist you in maintaining your power and perseverance throughout these procedures, as well as reminding you to take it easy on yourself if things go wrong. After all, you're only human!

Labradorite

This stone looks like a mix of all magical and ethereal colors that you could imagine swirling into forms within a piece of it. The many colors of this stone, particularly its blues and greens, demonstrate how it gives harmony to various Chakras, such as the neck and heart Chakras.

Labradorite amplifies your spiritual vibrations and connections. This implies that using it in meditations will often give you a much livelier experience and a piece of this rock under your pillow inspires colorful, insightful dreams at night.

Lapis Lazuli

The elevated vibrations of Lapis Lazuli create it a crystal that appeals to anyone who wants to fast track their intellectual development. Of course, there are no true shortcuts to enlightenment, but there are methods to increase your receptivity to divine advice and this stone is one such way.

This crystal encourages a straightforward mind, frankness and honesty in your communication. It enables you to link greater concepts and views with more simple rules of life and to see your physical and spiritual self as two halves of the same whole.

The places and places that create the unique colors and marki

Leopard-Skin Jasper

ngs of this gem assist in showing that we all have our styles and features. This stone and its vibrations help you to see that there is no shame in being who you are.

But, of course, doing so implies lots of mending and development—so, fortunately, this stone can help with that, too. It links the multiple points within you that will assist you break the bonds that hold you away from being your greatest self. But it also provides you the compassion you need to excuse yourself and all the others who might have wronged you along the manner.

Lepidolite

Lepidolite is correlated with development, but it also reminds us that advancement requires time. It's also sometimes awkward or depends on the old or obsolete being demolished or left behind.

The larger image is put into perspective when you operate with the healing fluids of Lepidolite. It will give you the power to take a step back and observe the course of life from afar and further, to take heart in the knowledge that any discomfort that you may encounter in your way today is only temporary.

Lepidolite enables you with all elements of conversion, including physical development, which means it's a nice dietary help or a fresh perspective.

CONCLUSION

Ibelieve that whatever is presented in this book is helpful to you. From natural healing methods to just have a general knowledge about crystals, I hope you learn the transformational power that crystals carry. Please have a notion that crystals can heal your body before you practise using crystals. A belief in crystals is must to understand its significant so that you can use its healing power to heal your body and to strengthen your immune system. The more you have a positive view of how the crystals work, the more it will have a positive impact on you.

If you understand this book, you will experience divination, the importance of meditation, and the meaning of pursuing a spiritual quest. At least, a little bit. If not, you are still possessed with having general knowledge about crystals, or if read properly, then an in-depth knowledge. It is very important to maintain a balance between the physical and emotional state of our body. It is important to understand our psychic abilities, the development of our intuition, and the overall health in general. If crystals can help in the holistic health of our body, reviving all the seven major chakras and the uncountable minor chakras in our body, there is nothing wrong with trying all the other methods that our science don't offer. Again, here there is no denying of modern medicine, but encouraging people to know all aspects of our nature, so that people can understand the world better.

Read this book thoroughly so that you can dive in the quest to understand and heal your body better. Understand the power that crystals through the millennia possessed and are still reigning today in the world where most advanced, affective ways had taken place to combat the diseases that attack the immune system. Understand how crystals help not only combating those diseases but doing spiritual work too to expand the potential of the human body. Don't neglect the power of crystals, believe in them so that they can believe in you. Get to know how the crystals work with chakras. Also, how crystals work with reiki. This book has all the necessary information that crystal lovers need. Happy healing!

www.ingramcontent.com/pod-product-compliance
Lightning Source LLC
Chambersburg PA
CBHW071824080526
44589CB00012B/910